MCQ Tutor In Anaesthesia: Clinical Practice

For Churchill Livingstone

Publisher: Geoffrey Nuttall
Project Editor: Lowri Daniels
Copy Editor: Joanna Smith
Production Controller: Neil Dickson
Sales Promotion Executive: Caroline Boyd

MCQ Tutor in Anaesthesia: Clinical Practice

Colin A. Pinnock
MB BS FRCAnaes
Consultant Anaesthetist, Alexandra Hospital, Redditch, UK

Robert M. Haden
MB ChB FRCAnaes
Consultant Anaesthetist, Alexandra Hospital, Redditch, UK

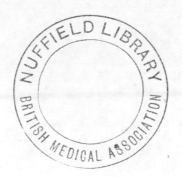

CHURCHILL LIVINGSTONE
EDINBURGH LONDON MADRID MELBOURNE NEW YORK AND TOKYO 1993

CHURCHILL LIVINGSTONE
Medical Division of Longman Group UK Limited

Distributed in the United States of America by Churchill
Livingstone Inc., 650 Avenue of the Americas, New York,
N.Y. 10011, and by associated companies, branches and
representatives throughout the world.

First published 1993

ISBN 0-443-04610-7

British Library Cataloguing in Publication Data
A catalogue record for this book is available from the
British Library.

Library of Congress Cataloging in Publication Data

Produced by Longman Singapore Publishers (Pte) Ltd.
Printed in Singapore

Contents

Preface

Candidates for the anaesthesia diploma examination have a seemingly insatiable appetite for multiple choice material. This volume sets out to satisfy some at least of that voracious appetite. It has been written in the same style as its sister volume *MCQ Tutor in Basic Sciences for Anaesthesia* which was intended for those candidates studying for the Part 2 FRCAnaes Diploma. This text is aimed at those attempting the final part of the examination. A similar approach has been retained for the layout. Questions number 270, equivalent to three 'mock' papers of 90 each. The discursive answers are referenced as before to sources of established expertise for the reader to consult when necessary. Whilst every effort has been made to use mostly those sources to which candidates have ready access (as detailed in David et al BJA (1900)64:6), it has often been necessary to stop into less well marked territory. The bibliography included at the back serves as an Index to the short reference titles used in the text.

The questions have been carefully arranged to give a good feel for the real situation. On occasions where ambiguity exists (and this is necessarily more marked with material on clinical situations), this is pointed out; occasionally the response given is the authors' choice and is clearly stated as such.

Introductory sections on the structure of the examination, both general and specific to the Part 3, have been included for the readers' benefit along with the 'How To Use' section and notes on MCQ technique. The pass rate in the final part of the FRCAnaes is somewhat greater than that for the Part 2 examination (around 40%). It is, nonetheless, not high. It is our hope that this modest volume will go some way to remedy this and it is in this spirit that this book is offered to the beleaguered candidate.

Our colleagues at the Alexandra Hospital have our grateful thanks for their support and encouragement over the last eighteen months.

Finally, our thanks are due to Dr P. V. Scott for his help with proof reading and to Dr R. P. Jones for the index.

Alexandra Hospital,
Redditch 1992

C. A. Pinnock
R. M. Haden

Acknowledgements

There are direct quotes from the following sources:

Question 11, Reference 11.1, BMJ (1976) 2 Diagnosis of Brain Death. Conference of the Medical Royal Colleges and Faculties of the United Kingdom, p1187

Question 12, Reference 12.1, Recommendations for Standards of Monitoring during Anaesthesia and Recovery. Association of Anaesthetists of Great Britain and Ireland 1988

A Guide to The Part 3 FRCAnaes Examination

THE FRCAnaes DIPLOMA

The three-part examination for the Diploma of Fellow of the Royal College of Anaesthetists is intended to test both depth of knowledge and application of that knowledge across the fields of anaesthesia covered in basic specialist training (BST). In brief these comprise general anaesthetic practice, intensive care medicine and the relief of chronic pain. The third part of this examination (Part 3 FRCAnaes) tests application of basic sciences to the practice of clinical anaesthesia.

AIMS OF THE PART 3 FRCAnaes

Candidates who achieve success in this section will already have gained a detailed knowledge of basic anaesthetic practice as tested in the Part 1 examination, and have a thorough grounding in the sciences of pharmacology and physiology as examined in the Part 2 examination. Success in the second part will demonstrate a sound and thorough grounding in the basic sciences which will enable progress to be made in clinical experience, leading to success in the final part of the examination and the attainment of the diploma itself.

THE SCOPE OF THE PART 3 FRCAnaes

Knowledge in the following broad areas is required prior to attempting the Part 3 FRCAnaes.

MEDICINE AND SURGERY

Those aspects which relate to pre-, intra- and postoperative management of patients and commonly occurring emergency situations, including intensive care management.

PREOPERATIVE PREPARATION

The taking of history and physical examination of patients. Knowledge of the impact of pathology on choice of anaesthetic and the preparation of the patient for surgery. Ventilation, general anaesthesia and intensive care medicine.

GENERAL ANAESTHESIA

Pharmacology of anaesthetic agents and their routes of administration. Physiological effects of anaesthesia. Anatomy of relevance. Clinical measurement related to anaesthesia and intensive care. Complications of anaesthesia and hazards associated with equipment. Monitoring equipment and its limitations, together with understanding and interpretation of data and sources of error therein.

General patient care under anaesthesia, including specific problems of any surgical procedure falling within basic specialist training (BST).

General principles of anaesthetic management of surgical procedures falling within higher specialist training (HST).

Acute pain relief. Morbidity and mortality and the principles of audit. The physical principles underlying the measurement of physiological variables with particular emphasis on functional testing of the cardiovascular, respiratory, neurological, renal and hepatic systems.

LOCAL ANAESTHESIA

Relevant anatomy, physiology and pharmacology. Equipment used, techniques, complications and indications.

POSTOPERATIVE MANAGEMENT

Monitoring and assessment in the recovery area. Early and late complications and their management. Care of the unconscious patient. The provision of analgesia.

INTENSIVE CARE MEDICINE

Pathophysiology of organ failure. Diagnostic procedures. Principles of management including fluid balance, sedation, organ support and analgesia. Nutritional support, infection control and sterilization of equipment.

Technology relevant to intensive care practice. Complications of intensive therapy, Severity scoring, ethical issues including brain stem death and organ transplantation.

RESUSCITATION

Assessment and management of cardiac and respiratory arrest. Emergency pacing. Resuscitation algorithms. Inter-hospital transfer of severely injured patients. Major disaster procedures.

SCIENTIFIC ASPECTS OF ANAESTHESIA AND INTENSIVE CARE

Developments and innovations featured in the major world literature. Critique of scientific papers. The design of clinical trials. Applications of computing to anaesthesia.

TRAUMA

Immediate management of the trauma victim, assessment and treatment of life-threatening situations. Triage. Airway management and artificial ventilatory support.

Hypovolaemic, cardiogenic and neurogenic shock and their treatment. Neurological assessment and scoring systems. Management of burns, Complications of treatment.

HISTORY

Although not regarded as essential, a knowledge of the history of anaesthesia is encouraged.

THE STRUCTURE OF THE PART 3 FRCAnaes EXAMINATION

The examination has five sections:
1. Written essay paper. Eight questions in two groups of four. Five questions must be answered, two from each group and a further question from either group. The time allowed is three hours.
2. MCQ paper. 90 questions. The time allowed is 160 min.
3. Clinical situation with patient. At present the clinical examination takes place with a single patient. Twenty five minutes are allotted to the taking of history and examination after which there is a period of 30 minutes with two examiners which may include other specimen material such as X-rays, ECG material, etc. unrelated to the patient. Currently the clinical examination is moving onto a different footing where candidates will be presented with a variety of clinical situations at 'stations'. The first of these, termed 'objectively structured clinical examination' (OSCE), has not yet been held. OSCE is likely to begin in 1994.
4. Oral examination with two examiners. The time allowed is 30 minutes.
5. Oral examination with two examiners. The time allowed is 30 minutes.

MARKING SYSTEM

A close marking system is used in all parts of the examination. The system is as follows:
2+ A good pass and very difficult to obtain!
2 A pass.
1+ A bare fail.
1 A bad fail.

Counselling is being introduced for candidates applying to take the examination for a fifth time. It is not yet clear whether this will be mandatory. Detailed information on all parts of the examination is available in the College publication entitled 'Guide to Training', May 1990. This is available on request from The Royal College of Anaesthetists, 48–49 Russell Square, London. Alternatively it can be obtained from local College Tutors.

Notes on MCQ Technique

Multiple choice question papers are designed to test factual recall. Throughout the three parts of the FRCAnaes the same multiple choice format is used. This consists of an interrogative or stem followed by five separate completions which may be marked true, false or don't know.

Candidates score +1 mark for each correct response and −1 for each incorrect response while don't know scores zero. In the examination, a question book is provided in which are the stems and completions and also a lector sheet on which to mark answer choices by way of pencilled bars. It is most strongly advised that answers are made in the question book before transferring them to the lector sheet. Be absolutely scrupulous in marking the lector sheet in accordance with your answers, as minor errors in numbering will prove disastrous. It is all too easy under stress to become confused.

Certain pitfalls deserve mention. Double check any question or part relating to opposites, for example hypo and hyper. If you get the sense reversed then minus five marks will result.

Beware of double negatives which needlessly confuse. While ideally there should not be any, in reality you will meet a few at least. Do not be overly suspicious of obvious false distractors. It is tempting to assume that if only you were more widely read then you would know of the connection between serum molybdenum and halothane hepatitis. Readers will be quick to spot that extensive reading is essential as a defence against this situation. Subjects which involve a great deal of controversy and debate may be best avoided for safety but there is an obvious limit to that particular gambit. There are remarkably few MCQ questions which are all true or all false but remember that these may occasionally occur. Be very suspicious of 'always' and 'never' in a stem. It is also difficult to put value judgements on 'frequently' and 'often'.

When MCQ papers are marked by computer, which is the commonest procedure, each of the completions is ascribed a facility index and a discrimination index. Put simply, the facility index is the proportion of candidates answering that particular atom correctly. It is an index of 'easiness'. In contrast, the discrimination index provides a measure of how well a particular stem will distinguish between good and bad candidates. This is obtained by choosing a proportion of good and bad candidates (for example the top and bottom 25%) and subtracting the number of correct answers in the lower category from those in the top. Hopefully a positive figure is obtained. In situations where the discrimination index is negative (in other words where more bad candidates scored highly than good ones) the completion needs examining for poor construction. Application of these indices will lead to an evolving higher standard of both stem and completion. Regrettably, the need for the introduction of new material on a regular basis requires the process to be continuous.

In summary, practical points to keep in the front of your mind as you confront the question paper are listed below for emphasis.

MOST IMPORTANT–DO NOT GUESS!
1.   READ EACH QUESTION VERY CAREFULLY.
2.   MAKE SURE THAT YOU FULLY UNDERSTAND IT.
3.   BE ESPECIALLY WARY OF QUESTIONS WITH OPPOSITES.
4.   DO NOT SPEND TOO MUCH TIME ON ANY ONE QUESTION.
5.   THINK CLEARLY AND DO NOT PANIC.
6.   DO NOT PURSUE THE ANSWER TOO FAR BUT RESPOND ONLY TO THE SIMPLE QUESTION WHICH HAS BEEN POSED.
7.   LEAVE SUFFICIENT TIME TO COMPLETE THE LECTOR SHEET.

How to Use the Book

The maximum benefit from using this book as a revision aid will be obtained if the basic reading has been completed first.

As you work through the book you will find on the left-hand page two questions each preceded by a short introduction. Below them on the same page are listed the references which are keyed to the answers. Each couplet of questions has the answers displayed on the right hand page.

It is suggested for revision that a sheet of paper or card is used to cover the answers while the questions are being attempted. Apart from concealing the answers, this sheet may be used to record your choices for each completion. If a question is encountered about which you know very little, use the references below to read around the subject before answering. This will enable you to make the most of the revision exercise.

The references are quoted in shortened form and most of them will be familiar. A complete list of the short references will be found in the bibliography at the back of the book. They are listed in full in alphabetical order and any unfamiliar source can be identified. Rather than being merely a list, the bibliography also gives some indication of the respective relevance of each text. Scanning it will indicate the scope of the reading necessary. Nearly all the texts are the currently available editions. Some older texts which have not been recently revised have been used where they are classic in nature and likely to be in every postgraduate library. An example of this is Davenport's famous text on acid-base balance (1974).

Finally, there is an index of subjects on page 285. Where a topic in the index is followed by a number alone, this indicates that the whole question is on that subject. In contrast, if a topic is followed by a number <u>and</u> a letter then it is the completion within a question which relates. For example, in the index '2, 3-DPG, 149d, 152' indicates that 2, 3-DPG is featured in question 149, completion d and is the main subject in question 152 to which all completions will refer. The index will enable the selection of any one particular topic for revision by indicating each and every occasion on which that topic occurs.

1 The haemoglobinopathies are pathological conditions in which there are disorders of haemoglobin synthesis which result in the inclusion of abnormal haemoglobin into red cells. One of the more frequently encountered haemoglobinopathies in clinical practice is sickle cell disease.

The following are true of sickle cell trait:
a) it is a homozygous state
b) it is inherited as a Mendelian dominant
c) it presents with severe anaemia
d) it will be detected by the Sickledex test
e) it may be diagnosed by electrophoresis

2 Massive blood transfusion has several definitions. Usually these incorporate total volume given and rate of transfusion per unit of blood. Here the definition may be taken as more than eight units of blood transfused, replacement of more than 40% of the blood volume or transfusion at a rate greater than a single unit in five minutes (2.5).

The following occur after massive transfusion of citrated blood:
a) metabolic acidosis
b) decreased plasma ionized calcium
c) hypokalaemia
d) hyponatraemia
e) hypothermia

References

1.1	Stoelting	p 567–568
1.2	Davidson	p 719–721
1.3	Churchill-Davidson	p 606
1.4	Synopsis	p 392–393
2.1	Synopsis	p 823–824
2.2	Transfusion	p 54
2.3	Transfusion	p 53
2.4	Scurr, Feldman & Soni	p 474
2.5	Miller	p 1473
2.6	Churchill-Davidson	p 597

1a) F Sickle trait is a heterozygous state in which up to 40% of the patient's haemoglobin is HbS, the remainder being HbA. The two forms are mixed in the same cell. Patients with the homozygous state have 95% haemoglobin HbS, a small proportion of HbF and no HbA (1.1).

  b) F A true Mendelian dominant would present with the full features of the condition in the heterozygous state. This is not so in sickle cell disease, which shows features of both dominant and recessive inheritance (1.2).

  c) F Patients with sickle cell <u>trait</u> may have a normal or slightly reduced haemoglobin concentration. It is sickle cell <u>anaemia</u> which presents with severe anaemia (except in the first three months of life, where HbF, the fetal variety, is the predominant form) (1.1, 1.3).

  d) T The Sickledex test shows a precipitate in the presence of HbS but cannot distinguish adequately between homozygous and heterozygous states (1.4).

  e) T Electrophoresis will reveal all the haemoglobin variants present and will therefore differentiate between trait and anaemia by showing the presence of both HbA and HbS (1.1).

2a) T Citrate is metabolized in the liver to bicarbonate. The capacity for this is large and can only be overwhelmed by rapid, large-scale transfusion which causes an initial metabolic acidosis, replaced later by alkalosis. The cells of the stored blood produce significant quantities of lactate and pyruvate, contributing to the initial acidosis (2.1, 2.2).

  b) T Citrate binds ionized calcium (the mechanism of its anticoagulant effect). Because citrate is quickly metabolized (see above) the binding is not usually a problem but it may become so after massive transfusion (2.1, 2.3,).

  c) F Effete cells in stored blood leak potassium. The plasma potassium concentration in stored blood may reach 30 mmol/l. There is a diluent effect in the general circulation but there will still be a rise in the recipient plasma concentration of potassium above its previous level. The effects of hyperkalaemia will be compounded by the hypocalcaemia caused by citrate (2.1, 2.3). Hypokalaemia would only occur after a massive transfusion of washed red cells where the potassium had been removed from the storage medium (2.5).

  d) F If the sodium–potassium cellular pump fails, as it must do for cellular leakage of potassium, there will also be leakage of sodium into the cell, reducing the extracellular concentration of sodium. However, the blood is stored in <u>sodium</u> citrate and the extracellular concentration of sodium starts at about 170 mmol/l on day one of storage, falling to about 155 mmol/l by day 28. The tendency is thus for the recipient to become <u>hyper</u>natraemic not <u>hypo</u>natraemic (2.4).

  e) T Blood is stored at 4°C. Large-scale transfusion of fluid at this temperature will reduce body temperature. Blood warmers may lessen this effect but they are still inefficient, especially at high flow rates (2.1, 2.2, 2.4, 2.6).

3 Dextrans are falling into disuse as plasma volume expanders because of the availability of less antigenic solutions. There are several dextran colutions each having different properties. The stem reads 'can occur' but does not specify a particular solution, so take care.

The following can occur after dextran infusion:
a) decreased coagulability
b) difficulties with cross matching
c) renal tubular damage
d) rouleaux formation
e) anaphylactoid reactions

4 Electrolytes and fluid balance are favourite topics in Part 3 FRCAnaes. The clinical states described in such questions are not uncommon in clinical practice, though their relative importance is another matter.

In a state of water retention the following abnormalities may occur:
a) low serum sodium
b) low urine output
c) increased right atrial pressure
d) increased body weight
e) tachycardia

References

3.1	Vickers, Morgan & Spencer	p 504
3.2	Data Sheet Compendium	p 1342
3.3	Synopsis	p 826
3.4	Churchill-Davidson	p 590–591
3.5	Dundee, Clarke & McCaughey	p 551–552
4.1	Churchill-Davidson	p 581
4.2	Churchill-Davidson	p 572
4.3	Synopsis	p 482
4.4	Stoelting	p 451–453

3a) T Dextran 70 (average molecular weight 70 000 daltons) has been used for the prophylaxis of deep vein thrombosis because of its effects on coagulation, especially those of reducing platelet aggregation and altering the chemical stability of fibrin. These effects are properties of the dextran molecule itself rather than molecular weight, although Dextran 40 is said not to have this effect. Confusingly, dextrans are also said to increase platelet stickiness (3.1, 3.2).

b) T Cross matching is compromised by the coating of red cells, which alters the electrical charge on the cell membrane and therefore prevents aggregation under laboratory conditions unless the cells are washed first. Dextran 40 does not interfere with cross matching. References are contradictory but (3.3) is especially informative (3.1, 3.2, 3.3).

c) T Dextran 40 especially, being largely excreted in the urine, produces tubular fluid with a high viscosity which causes high renal tubular pressure and reversible renal dysfunction (3.1, 3.4).

d) T Rouleaux formation occurs and may contribute to difficulties in cross matching with Dextran 70 but not with Dextran 40 (3.3).

e) T The dextrans have a low incidence of anaphylactoid response (0.008% for severe reactions). Release of histamine in an anaphylactoid manner is implicated in these although a haptogenic role is the likely cause of life-threatening reactions (3.5).

4a) T Low serum sodium concentration is one of the cardinal signs of water excess, from whatever cause. It is most commonly seen after transurethral prostatectomy (TUR syndrome). There are also conditions where low serum sodium concentration is a result of sodium loss but these are far less common than water excess (4.1, 4.2, 4.3).

b) T Renal disease may cause water retention. If renal function was previously normal the urine output may still be low because of oedema of the renal medulla. Urine output in water retention states will usually be low (4.4).

c) T Water excess and the associated hyponatraemia imply a high intravascular volume and therefore a high right atrial pressure. The effect of hyponatraemia on myocardial contractility will exaggerate this effect (4.4).

d) T This completion speaks for itself. Repeated weighing can be used to assess progress in the treatment of the condition (4.4).

e) F Interstitial oedema caused by water retention causes a fall in myocardial electrical activity and contractility which results in a fall in cardiac rate (4.4).

5 Questions which incorporate biochemical values can be infuriating. The values given rarely fit into a definite pattern, but the stem usually says 'are compatible with' rather than 'diagnostic of'.

Serum biochemical values (mmol/l) sodium 127, potassium 6.0, urea 18, glucose 3, bicarbonate 18 are compatible with:
a) renal failure
b) Addison's disease
c) inappropriate secretion of antidiuretic hormone
d) hepatic failure
e) fluid overload

6 Cardiac tamponade is characterized by reduced stroke volume and arterial pressure due to raised intrapericardial pressure. The causes of accumulation of pericardial fluid are diverse.

The following are true of acute cardiac tamponade:
a) it can be associated with aortic dissection
b) the JVP is low and falls further on inspiration
c) the radial artery blood pressure falls on expiration
d) diuretics are preferred to paracentesis as first line treatment
e) the presence of hepatomegaly would suggest right heart failure rather than tamponade

References

5.1	Dunnill & Colvin	p 73–76
5.2	Stoelting	p 420–425
5.3	Davidson	p 650–651
5.4	Whitby, Smith & Beckett	p 49–50
5.5	Zilva & Pannall	p 46–55
6.1	Souhami & Moxham	p 434
6.2	OTM	p 14.8–9
6.3	OTM	p 14.12
6.4	OTM	p 13.308–309
6.5	OTM	p 12.273

5 Normal serum values (mmol/l) are. Sodium 135–148, Potassium 3.8–5.0, Urea 2.5–6.5, Glucose 3.0–4.6, Bicarbonate 24–32 (5.1).

a) **T** The term 'renal failure' covers a multitude of conditions, all of which tend to cause acidosis, hyperkalaemia and uraemia along with dilutional hyponatraemia. This pattern is marked in pre-renal failure and the oliguric phase of acute renal failure (5.2).

b) **T** During Addisonian crisis, sodium loss exceeds water loss, causing hyponatraemia with hyperkalaemia and metabolic acidosis. The fluid depletion then causes a reduction in renal function with a moderate rise in serum urea. The chronic Addisonian state shows serum sodium concentration in the low normal range (5.3).

c) **F** Inappropriate ADH secretion causes dilutional effects on all blood values. The high potassium and urea values here suggest that this is not the case (5.4).

d) **F** Hepatic failure produces a secondary hyperaldosteronism which results in hyponatraemia, (although whole body sodium is increased), normal or low potassium values and low urea with oedema because of reduced plasma proteins. Serum urea concentration is thus reduced by both dilution and depressed production (5.5).

e) **F** Fluid overload will produce a dilutional hypokalaemia and low serum urea as seen in inappropriate ADH secretion (5.4).

6a) **T** The aortic root lies within the pericardium and so aortic root dissection may perforate retrogradely into the pericardium (0.1, 0.2).

b) **F** In tamponade, the heart can empty but not fill. The JVP will be high and increase further on inspiration (6.2, 6.3).

c) **F** Pulsus paradoxus is one of the cardinal signs of tamponade, though in fact there is nothing paradoxical about it. It is merely a gross extension of the normal respiratory swing in blood pressure. This results in a fall in blood pressure on inspiration (6.2).

d) **F** Tamponade is a life-threatening emergency. The treatment is paracentesis (pericardial tap). Diuretics have no place. If the situation is not desperate enough to warrant paracentesis then the diagnosis is wrong (6.2, 6.3).

e) **T** The hepatomegaly of right heart failure is the result of chronic venous congestion. In tamponade there is insufficient time for the liver to become enlarged (6.4, 6.5).

7 Hyperkalaemia is a common clinical problem which may result from renal impairment, transfusion, burns, trauma, among other causes.

In hyperkalaemia:
a) there is a tall, peaked T wave
b) there is a U wave
c) there is a deep S wave
d) ventricular fibrillation may occur
e) digoxin toxicity may be potentiated

8 Difficult endotracheal intubation is often unpredictable. There are, however, a number of conditions where it may be anticipated and therefore dealt with with less morbidity and more control.

Difficult endotracheal intubation may be anticipated in:
a) Treacher–Collins syndrome
b) Pierre Robin syndrome
c) Klippel–Feil syndrome
d) Shy–Drager syndrome
e) Sturge–Weber syndrome

References

7.1	Rowlands 2	p 225–226
7.2	Dundee, Clarke & McCaughey	p 590–591
8.1	Katz & Kadis	p 689
8.2	Katz & Kadis	p 582
8.3	Anesthesiology (1971); 35:	p 95–97
8.4	Stoelting	p 308–309

7 It is essential for a clinical anaesthetist to be able to manage the problems of hyperkalaemia, whatever the cause. The most commonly asked causes are trauma, burns, the use of suxamethonium and renal failure.
   a) T A tall, peaked T wave is the classic ECG change of hyperkalaemia. The plasma concentrations at which this occurs may vary, but will usually be above 5.5 mmol/l (7.1).
   b) F The U wave is a sign of hypokalaemia rather than hyperkalaemia (7.1).
   c) F Hyperkalaemia tends, above a plasma concentration of 6.5 mmol/l, to cause depression or elevation of the ST segment rather than an S wave per se (7.1).
   d) T Ventricular fibrillation is the ultimate result of gross hyperkalaemia, occurring above a plasma concentration of about 7.5 mmol/l (7.1).
   e) F Hyperkalaemia does not potentiate the effects of digoxin toxicity but hypokalaemia will (7.2).

8 Although 'syndrome spotting' tends to be a medical pastime rather than an anaesthetic one, there are some syndromes which should trigger interest and further investigation because of their major implications for the conduct of anaesthesia and the safety of the patient.
   a) T Treacher–Collins syndrome is characterized by choanal atresia, ophthalmic abnormalities and congenital heart defects as well as the hypoplasia of the facial and jaw bones which is of relevance to intubation (8.1).
   b) T Pierre Robin syndrome presents as micrognathia, macroglossia and cleft palate. The tongue may be placed further back than usual in the airway, compounding airway difficulties. In the neonate the airway can often only be maintained by the use of a tongue stitch (8.1).
   c) T In Klippel–Feil syndrome the cervical vertebrae fail to differentiate. The most common form is fusion of C2 and C3 though the whole cervical spine and occiput may be involved. The neck is usually short overall. There are also thoracic abnormalities which may interfere with ventilation (spontaneous or controlled) under anaesthesia (8.2).
   d) F Although Shy–Drager syndrome does not lead to airway or intubation problems, it is of interest because of the variable degree of autonomic failure which leads to difficulties with cardiovascular stability. Theoretically it would seem logical to use epidural or spinal anaesthesia in these patients because they are already maximally vasodilated. Unfortunately there is a distinct lack of reference material and that which exists suggests that cardiovascular stability is no better using regional anaesthesia than general. Most sources refer to Cohen (8.3) yet fail to emphasize that the regional block in that particular case report failed to work (8.2, 8.3).
   e) F Patients with the features of Sturge–Weber syndrome have angiomatous abnormalities about the upper face and head and in the brain. There are no consistent airway or intubation problems (8.4).

9 Reference texts and journals have a habit of using several different systems of measurement. For example, the SI unit of pressure is N/m^2 but medical texts use a mixture of mmHg, kPa and cmH_2O.

A normal value for atmospheric pressure at sea level would be:
a) 760 mmHg
b) 10350 cmH_2O
c) 14.7 lb/in^2
d) 101.33 N/m^2
e) 101.33 kPa

10 The practice of regional anaesthesia demands a detailed knowledge of neuroanatomy.

The trigeminal nerve supplies:
a) the mucosa of the soft palate
b) the tympanic membrane
c) the skin over the angle of the mandible
d) the ala nasae
e) the conjunctiva

References

9.1 Dunnill & Colvin   p 233–236

10.1 Gray   p 1289
10.2 Gray   p 1104
10.3 Gray   p 1106
10.4 Gray   p 1216

9 This is a simple matter of factual recall. A Newton is the unit of force which will give a 1 kg mass an acceleration of 1 m/s^2. It is advisable to be able to convert between units: 1 mmHg = 1.36 cmH$_2$O = 133.3 N/m^2 = 0.0194 psi = 0.133 kPa. Thus, one atmosphere absolute may also be expressed as: 14.7 psi, 29.9 mmHg, 1035 cmH$_2$O, 101.33 kPa, 1.0133 x 10^5 N/m^2 or 1 bar! (9.1).

a) T
b) T
c) T
d) F
e) T

10a) T Via the greater and lesser palatine branches of the mandibular division of the trigeminal nerve (10.1).
 b) T Via the auriculotemporal branch of the posterior trunk of the mandibular division of the trigeminal nerve (10.2).
 c) F The skin overlying the angle of the mandible is supplied by the greater auricular nerve which is formed from cervical roots 2 and 3 (10.3).
 d) T Via the maxillary division of the trigeminal (10.3).
 e) T Via the ophthalmic division of the trigeminal nerve (10.4).

11 The preconditions and tests for brain stem death are essential knowledge. Be prepared to provide them at short notice.

The following are each part of the diagnostic criteria for the establishment of 'brain stem death' recommended for use in Britain by the Conference of Medical Royal Colleges and Faculties of the UK:
a) one of the two certifying doctors must be a specialist neurologist
b) the cause of the coma need not be established if recovery seems unlikely
c) the pupils must be dilated, equal in size and unresponsive to sudden changes in the intensity of incident light
d) a core temperature below 35 °C invalidates testing
e) the return of spinal reflexes after a period of absence invalidates testing

12 Keeping up to date with current trends and recommendations is important. The document to which this question refers is required reading.

The Association of Anaesthetists of Great Britain and Ireland 'Recommendations for Standards of Monitoring during Anaesthesia and Recovery' states:
a) whenever neuromuscular blocking agents are in use, a peripheral nerve stimulator must be used
b) sedative and local anaesthetic techniques are excluded from the recommendations
c) an oxygen concentration monitor must always be used in the patient breathing system
d) the use of a device to prevent the administration of hypoxic mixtures is recommended
e) capnography is not considered necessary in spontaneously breathing patients

References

11.1 BMJ (1976) 2 p 1187
Diagnosis of Brain Death. Conference of the Medical Royal Colleges and Faculties of the United Kingdom.

12.1 Recommendations for Standards of Monitoring during Anaesthesia and Recovery. Association of Anaesthetists of Great Britain and Ireland 1988.

11 The most important elements of the criteria for the diagnosis of brain stem death are the preconditions and exclusions. There was media hysteria in the late 1970s because cases were presented as 'recovery after being diagnosed brain dead' when the preconditions had not even been considered. The tests mean nothing without both a solid diagnosis for the cause of coma and very careful exclusion of pharmacological and biochemical contributions.

a) F The criteria make no recommendations as to grade or specialty of the clinicians involved in the testing except to say that there should be two of them and that they should have experience in the management of such cases.

b) F 'There should be no doubt that the patient's condition is due to irremediable structural brain damage. The diagnosis of a disorder which can lead to brain death should have been fully established.'

c) T 'The pupils are fixed in diameter and do not respond to sharp changes in the intensity of incident light.'

d) F 'Primary hypothermia as a cause of coma should have been excluded.' The patient should have had a normal temperature at some stage of their admission.

e) F 'It is well established that spinal cord function can persist after insults which irretrievably destroy brain function. Reflexes of spinal origin may persist or return after an initial absence in brain dead patients.'

12 The Association's recommendations are not mandatory. Even so, it is very difficult to justify ignoring recommendations from professional bodies (12.1).

a) F 'should be readily available' not compulsory.

b) F 'the same considerations apply to any local or regional anaesthetic technique or sedation involving the risk of unconsciousness'.

c) T The recommendation is that the oxygen concentration delivered to the patient should always be monitored. This implies that there should be an oxygen monitor in the breathing system.

d) F The recommendation is that the oxygen concentration delivered to the patient should be monitored and have an alarm. There is no recommendation that this should be interlinked to the flowmeters to prevent the administration of hypoxic mixtures, but more machines are being manufactured to include this feature.

e) F 'carbon dioxide tracing should be used... during both mechanical and spontaneous ventilation'.

13 The Part 3 FRCAnaes includes a large element of physics and clinical measurement.

When gas flows through a tube:
a) laminar flow implies that flow is smooth and parallel to the walls of the tube
b) with laminar flow, resistance is directly proportional to the diameter of the tube
c) above the critical flow rate, turbulent flow results
d) at a constriction, sharp curve or valve, turbulent flow develops
e) when turbulent flow develops, flow is inversely proportional to the square of the gas density

14 Anaesthesia in the presence of both congenital and acquired heart disease is not confined to the correction of these defects. Draw on anatomical knowledge to help.

Air embolism is especially dangerous in:
a) atrial septal defect (ASD)
b) persistent ductus arteriosus (PDA)
c) ventricular septal defect (VSD)
d) aortic valve stenosis
e) pulmonary valve stenosis

References

| **13.1** Scurr, Feldman & Soni | p 33–36 |

| **14.1** Nimmo & Smith | p 599–600 |
| **14.2** Miller | p 1486 |

13 Laminar flow can only occur during flow along smooth-walled tubes without bends, acute corners or constrictions and below the critical flow rate. Outside these conditions Reynolds' number is exceeded and turbulent flow results.
  a) T Laminar flow is by definition smooth and occurs parallel to the walls of a cylinder (13.1).
  b) F Resistance is directly proportional to the fourth power of the radius (13.1).
  c) T The critical flow rate is related to Reynolds' number (13.1).
  d) T Laminar flow only holds for parallel sided vessels (13.1).
  e) F The transition from laminar to turbulent flow depends upon the relationship:

$$\text{critical velocity} = \frac{(2000 \times \text{viscosity})}{(\text{diameter} \times \text{density})}$$

  and therefore flow is inversely proportional to the density, not to its square (13.1).

14 Although any intracardiac shunt (and this includes patent ductus arteriosus) will have a potential for right-to-left transfer of air bubbles, the left sided pressures are usually higher than the right and so mitigate against this. References in many major texts contradict themselves in just this way. The danger of air embolus is threefold: in its prevention of cardiac emptying by foaming in the atrium or ventricle; in occlusion of the pulmonary circulation; and in the systemic effect of arterial occlusion, especially in the brain or other major organ. It is only the latter effect which is relevant here.
  a) T Air may pass through the ASD from right side to left (14.1, 14.2).
  b) T Air may pass through a patent ductus from pulmonary artery to aorta (14.1, 14.2).
  c) T Air may pass from right to left ventricle (14.1, 14.2).
  d) F In aortic stenosis there is no intracardiac shunt for the passage of air into the systemic circulation.
  e) F There is no reason why valve stenoses should make air embolism especially hazardous (see above).

15 Biochemistry of limited clinical significance. The specific wording of the stem requires careful consideration.

A state of low serum sodium and low total body sodium can occur in:
a) heart failure with oedema
b) renal failure
c) hepatocellular failure
d) water intoxication
e) inappropriate secretion of antidiuretic hormone

16 The physics of gas flow and measurement is directly relevant to the everyday practice of anaesthesia.

With respect to the measurement of gas flow:
a) the rotating bobbin is an example of a constant orifice device
b) the Fleisch pneumotachograph is an example of a variable orifice flowmeter
c) gases which have the same density will give similar readings in a rotating bobbin flowmeter
d) increasing the back pressure on a rotating bobbin flowmeter means that at a given indicated flow there will be an increased number of gas molecules passing per minute
e) at the narrowest part of a Venturi the pressure of gas will fall

References

15.1 Davidson   p 286–289
15.2 Whitby, Smith & Beckett   p 48–49
15.3 Zilva & Pannall   p 104

16.1 Scurr, Feldman & Soni   p 104–115
16.2 Ward   p 17

15a) F In cardiac failure with oedema there is both sodium and water retention which leads to a dilutional hyponatraemia with an increased total body sodium (15.1).

b) T In the diuretic phase of renal failure, a massive loss of sodium in the urine occurs leading to both hyponatraemia and low total body sodium. This is not the only condition where this pattern may occur. Recent ileostomy and major diarrhoea are similar sodium-losing conditions (15.2).

c) F The secondary hyperaldosteronism of hepatic failure leads to both sodium and water retention, water more than the sodium (15.3).

d) F In water intoxication there has been no loss of sodium although there may be a dilutional hyponatraemia (15.2).

e) F Sodium and water retention occurs in inappropriate ADH secretion, leading to increased total body sodium (15.1, 15.2).

16 The rotating bobbin is still the standard method of gas flow measurement on anaesthetic machines, and the pneumotachograph is a common means of flow measurement in anaesthetic and intensive care ventilators. The Venturi is used as a method of gas entrainment in oxygen therapy.

a) F The rotameter is an example of a variable orifice device, the orifice being annular around the bobbin and the outside diameter of the annulus increasing as the bobbin rises up the flowmeter tube (16.1).

b) F The pneumotachograph is a set of tubes or a meshwork which behaves as multiple Venturi orifices which cause a flow-dependent difference in pressure between the upstream and downstream sides. These orifices are constant (16.1).

c) F The flow of a gas through a constriction depends upon both density and viscosity. In general, if the constriction is an orifice then density plays the more important role, if the constriction is tubular then viscosity is more important. In a rotating bobbin the constriction is more tubular at low flows and more like an orifice at higher flows, therefore gases with the same density but different viscosities will behave differently at high and low flows and the readings will not correspond (16.1).

d) T Read the question very carefully. The indicated flow and the actual flow will be different because of back pressure. At a given indicated flow there will be a greater actual flow, i.e., a greater number of molecules passing per minute (16.1).

e) T This completion describes the working principle of the Venturi which is used to produce entrainment in oxygen supply devices (16.2).

17 ECG morphology requires revision. Ensure that the basic diagnostic criteria for each of the common rhythm abnormalities are known.

P waves are absent in:
a) atrial fibrillation
b) atrial flutter
c) nodal tachycardia
d) ventricular tachycardia
e) first degree heart block

18 The use of pulmonary artery flotation catheters has increased in recent years in both intensive care and operating theatre environments. It is common to receive one in the viva examination for discussion.

The pulmonary artery wedge pressure:
a) measures the right atrial pressure
b) reflects the left atrial pressure
c) is named from the wedge-shaped end of the catheter
d) is normally greater than 10 mmHg
e) is raised in tricuspid stenosis

References

17.1	Rowlands 3	p 431–436
17.2	Rowlands 3	p 459
17.3	Rowlands 3	p 461
17.4	Rowlands 3	p 488
18.1	Souhami & Moxham	p 545
18.2	Dunnill & Colvin	p 115

17a) T In atrial fibrillation there is disorganized atrial activity but no P waves (17.1).

b) F In atrial flutter there is atrial tachycardia such that there is no time for the electrical activity to return to baseline. This results in the classical 'sawtooth' pattern. The atrial rate is usually in the region of 250 beats/min or more (17.1).

c) F There is atrial activity in nodal rhythm but the P waves are hidden in the QRS complex. This begs the question of whether P waves are present if you cannot find them! (17.2).

d) F In ventricular tachycardia there is a re-entrant ventricular pattern independent of the atria. The atrial activity continues as normal. The P waves are hidden within the QRS but can usually be seen as voltage variations in the ventricular complexes (17.3).

e) F The definition of first degree heart block states that there are P waves but that they are separated from the QRS complex by more than 0.21 seconds (17.4).

18 The pulmonary artery catheter comes in a number of varieties, all designed for different purposes. The basic catheter for the measurement of pulmonary wedge pressure has only one lumen and a balloon. The balloon is inflated to float the catheter into the pulmonary artery and to float the tip of the catheter into a small vessel, occluding it proximally but not distally, preventing the passage of pulmonary arterial pressure waves past the balloon. This is the 'wedged' position. This manoeuvre leaves the vessel open distally through the capillaries into the pulmonary veins and the left atrium, and theory states that the pressure in the left atrium will equilibrate with that in the occluded vessel distal to the catheter. This can then be measured through the lumen of the catheter.

a) F The tip of the catheter is in a small pulmonary vessel, not in the right atrium (18.1).

b) T 'Reflects' is the operative word. Because of the vessels distal to the catheter tip, the wedged pressure does not give a direct left atrial pressure. To obtain a true left atrial pressure a catheter must be placed directly at operation or passed retrogradely from a systemic artery via the left ventricle (18.1).

c) F The name comes from the fact that the catheter is 'wedged' in a branch of the pulmonary artery, not from the shape of the catheter tip (18.1).

d) F The correct range is 6–12 mmHg rather than 'greater than 10' (18.2).

e) F The tricuspid valve lies between the right atrium and ventricle. Tricuspid stenosis will cause a high right atrial pressure with restricted onward movement of blood into the pulmonary and left-sided cardiac circulation. There will be disparity between the performance of the right and left sides of the heart. The CVP and the left atrial pressure will not be directly related. The PCWP will not be raised (18.1).

19 Physical properties of anaesthetic agents determine some of their effects and the differences between agents. A comparative chart makes a useful revision aid.

The blood/gas partition coefficient for an inhalational agent:
a) defines the solubility of the agent in blood
b) defines the potency of an agent
c) is related to the potency: the lower the partition coefficient, the greater is the potency.
d) is 12 for halothane
e) is 0.47 for nitrous oxide

20 Read the question carefully. Blood/gas and oil/gas partition coefficients are not the same.

The following are correct oil/gas partition coefficients:
a) nitrous oxide 1.4
b) halothane 422
c) enflurane 98.5
d) isoflurane 168
e) desflurane 19

References
19.1 Scurr, Feldman & Soni   p 576
19.2 Rang & Dale   p 606–614
19.3 Dunnill & Colvin   p 7

20.1 Rang & Dale   p 614
20.2 Scurr, Feldman & Soni   p 574
20.3 BJA (1990) 65   p 527–536

19a) F Solubility relates to the quantity of agent that can be dissolved in a given quantity of fluid, rather than to the partition coefficient which is the ratio of the amount in the gaseous phase compared to the fluid phase (19.1).

b) F BEWARE! There is more than one view of the meaning of 'potency' when applied to inhaled agents. It can be taken to mean either the speed of induction or the depth achievable. The first would mean that nitrous oxide would be highly potent, but the second would mean only weak potency because great depth is not achievable (hence a minimum alveolar concentration of greater than 100%). The accepted view is the second which is a reflection of MAC value – the only true way of comparing pharmacological potency between vapours. If this is so, then it is the oil/gas partition coefficient, as an indication of the fat solubility, which reflects potency, rather than the blood/gas coefficient (19.2).

c) F The speed of induction is determined by the blood/gas partition coefficient, not the 'potency' by the definition used above. Certainly, the less soluble (lower blood/gas partition coefficient) agents will give a more rapid induction (19.2).

d) F The value for halothane is 2.5. 12 relates to diethyl ether (19.3).

e) T (19.3).

20 The oil/gas partition coefficient relates to 'potency' (see above). Different sources tend to give slightly different results, but this is not of any great importance. See Table 1

a) T (20.1, 20.2).

b) F (20.1, 20.2).

c) T (20.1, 20.2).

d) F (20.2).

e) T (20.3).

Table 1 Oil/gas Partition coefficients from various sources

Source	A	B	C
Nitrous oxide	1.4	1.4	1.4
Halothane	220	224	224
Enflurane	98	98	96
Isoflurane	98	–	91
Desflurane	–	–	19
Sevoflurane	–	–	53
Cyclopropane	11.5	12	–
Trichlorethylene	–	714	–
Diethyl ether	65	65	–
Methoxyflurane	950	970	–

A Rang & Dale; B Scurr, Feldman & Soni; C BJA (1990) 65 p 527–536

21 The physics of solutions, solvents, solutes and partial pressures of gases have major implications in anaesthesia. The gas laws are basic secondary school physics.

Henry's law:
a) refers to the effect of volume on the temperature of a gas
b) states that the molecular force of a gas will be constant at constant pressure
c) refers to the concentration of a dissolved gas in a given solvent
d) assumes constant temperature
e) relates the concentration of a dissolved gas to its partial pressure

22 The effects of congenital heart disease upon anaesthesia and anaesthetic technique apply not only to cardiac surgical units but to incidental surgery in the patient with heart disease. Fallot's Tetralogy is the most common form of cyanotic congenital heart disease.

The Tetralogy of Fallot exhibits the following features:
a) pulmonary valve stenosis
b) atrial septal defect
c) right ventricular hypertrophy
d) the aorta overrides the right ventricle
e) patent ductus arteriosus

References

21.1 Scurr, Feldman & Soni   p 29
21.2 Scurr, Feldman & Soni   p 23–24

22.1 Churchill-Davidson   p 502–503

21 Henry's law states: 'The mass of a gas dissolved by a given volume of solvent, at a given constant temperature is proportional to the partial pressure of the gas in equilibrium with the solution' (21.1).

a) **F** It is not Henry's law but Charles' law which relates the temperature of a gas to its volume (21.2).

b) **F** This statement approximates to Boltzmann's constant, which includes a variable for temperature (21.2).

c) **T** As described above (21.1).

d) **T** 'A constant, given temperature' (21.1).

e) **T** In the manner described above. The greater the partial pressure, the more gas will dissolve (21.1).

22 The Tetralogy of Fallot has, as the name suggests, four basic features: pulmonary stenosis, right ventricular hypertrophy, ventricular septal defect and overriding aorta (22.1). There may occasionally be other associated features.

a) **F** The pulmonary stenosis is usually infundibular in nature (22.1).

b) **F** Atrial septal defect is not a feature of Fallot's Tetralogy (22.1).

c) **T** Right ventricular hypertrophy is seen, presumably because of the pulmonary stenosis (22.1).

d) **T** An overriding aorta is a variably anatomical feature, the clinical significance of which may not be great (22.1).

e) **F** Patent ductus arteriosus is not a regular feature of Fallot's Tetralogy (22.1).

23 Although the more recently introduced muscle relaxants, vecuronium and atracurium predominate in current practice (see SOAP), the older relaxants are still commonly used and should be included in revision.

Curare (*d*-tubocurarine):
a) causes a fall in blood pressure by ganglion blockade
b) is effective orally
c) was introduced into clinical practice by Magill in the 1930s
d) has a mild vagolytic effect
e) is excreted unchanged by the kidneys

24 **Pancuronium:**
a) is a steroid molecule
b) is highly bound to plasma albumin
c) is excreted unchanged in the bile
d) was introduced into clinical practice in the 1940's
e) reduces the MAC of halothane

References

23.1	Synopsis	p 255–257
23.2	Rang & Dale	p 166
23.3	Recent Advances 15	p 22
23.4	Rang & Dale	p 164
23.5	Rang & Dale	p 170
24.1	Recent Advances 15	p 22
24.2	Calvey & Williams	p 282–283
24.3	Vickers, Morgan & Spencer	p 267–269
24.4	Synopsis	p 270
24.5	Synopsis	p 256
24.6	Recent Advances 15	p 3

23 Curare was the first nondepolarizing neuromuscular blocker introduced into clinical anaesthesia, by Griffiths and Johnson in Canada in 1942 (23.1), having been a physiological curiosity since it was brought from South America in the 16th century.

a) **F** One of the myths of anaesthesia, handed down from generation to generation. In the doses usually used, around 0.5 mg/kg, the fall in blood pressure follows a dose-response curve to histamine. The ganglion blockade which occurs only becomes significant at higher doses (23.2, 23.3).

b) **F** Absorption from mucosal surfaces is slow, as would be expected from a highly ionized and poorly lipid-soluble drug. As a result it is ineffective by mouth (23.4). Significant oral absorption would have been embarrassing if animals were eaten uncooked after being killed by arrows tipped with curare!

c) **F** As described above (23.1).

d) **F** Such reference material as is available suggests that the vagolytic effect of curare is nil or minimal. Nil is the authors' preference here (23.3).

e) **T** Curare is excreted unchanged by the kidneys, but only 30–40% of a given dose is recoverable in this manner (23.5).

24 As can be readily seen from the size of the reference list, there is still a certain amount of controversy about pancuronium, despite its being in regular clinical use for 30 years.

a) **T** The pancuronium molecule has a steroid ring in it yet has no hormonal activity (24.1).

b) **F** Controversial. References vary in the quantification of protein binding and to which group of proteins. It seems that 70–80% of a given dose is protein bound, mostly to globulins, less to albumin. In clinical states where there is disturbance of the quantities or balance between the various groups of protein, there seems to be very little effect upon the intensity or duration of the neuromuscular blockade produced by pancuronium (24.2, 24.3, 24.4).

c) **T** Although excreted unchanged in the bile, 25% of a dose of pancuronium is first metabolized, to 3-hydroxy, 17-hydroxy and 3,17-hydroxy derivatives, the first of which is active at about half the potency of the parent drug (24.2, 24.4).

d) **F** See above (24.5).

e) **T** The mechanism behind this phenomenon is not clear, but it exists and is measurable (24.6).

25 The physical attributes of the anaesthetic vapours determine, to a large extent, their clinical characteristics. Saturated vapour pressure is a determinant of delivered concentration which, in conjunction with the other physical properties, will determine speed of induction and potency.

The following are correct saturated vapour pressures at 20°C:
a) ether 440 mmHg
b) halothane 241 mmHg
c) methoxyflurane 23 mmHg
d) enflurane 360 mmHg
e) trichlorethylene 636 mmHg

26 Malignant hyperpyrexia (MH) is fortunately rare. It is, however, one of the conditions which are of vital importance to the anaesthetist. Though seldom met in practice, MH is often encountered in examinations.

Malignant hyperpyrexia:
a) will not be triggered by the use of isoflurane
b) may be triggered by the amide local anaesthetics
c) must be suspected if the jaw fails to relax after suxamethonium
d) is inherited as a sex-linked recessive
e) was first reported from Australia in 1960

References

25.1	Churchill-Davidson	p 170
25.2	Vickers, Morgan & Spencer	p 124
25.3	Dunnill & Colvin	p 7
25.4	Synopsis	p 172
26.1	Recent Advances 15	p 173–207
26.2	BJA (1991) 67	p 515–516

25 Standard physical constants for the various anaesthetic gases and vapours are essential knowledge. There are some minor inconsistencies from text to text. See Table 2.
a) T
b) T
c) T
d) F
e) F

26 Malignant hyperpyrexia is an hereditary condition of skeletal muscle, inherited as an autosomal dominant with variable penetrance. Biochemical tests are not yet specific enough for routine preoperative screening.

   The main characteristics are that upon exposure to adequate doses of the depolarizing muscle relaxants or anaesthetic gases and vapours, there is a chaotic increase in muscle metabolism, resulting in spasm, gross acidosis, massive oxygen consumption and a rise in body temperature of more than 2°C per hour until treatment takes control or the patient dies with denatured proteins. It carries a 40–50% mortality in the acute event. For a full review see (26.1).

a) **F** All of the anaesthetic vapours are implicated, including the newer ones. There have been a number of cases reported where isoflurane was implicated. It seems that even sevoflurane is suspect, but only in pigs as yet (26.1).

b) **F** It is often said that amides can trigger MH, but there is evidence that even infusions of bupivacaine do not trigger susceptible pigs. Epidural anaesthesia with bupivacaine is recommended as an alternative to general anaesthesia (26.1).

c) **F** There has been a long debate on this very subject. The outcome is that there is a difference between spasm and failure to relax. The latter may more often be the result of a deterioration in the activity of the drug because of poor storage conditions (26.1, 26.2).

d) **F** The whole family must be investigated if there is one member in whom MH is triggered (26.1).

e) **T** Denborough reported in 1960 that a family had presented to him, several of whom had died under general anaesthesia. These were the first recognized cases, although they cannot have been the first deaths (26.1).

Table 2   Saturated vapour pressures according to various sources (mmHg at 20°C)

Source	A	B	C	D
Diethyl ether	440	442	425	425
Halothane	243	243.3	243	243
Methoxyflurane	22.5	23	25	–
Enflurane	184	184	180	174.5
Isoflurane	250	250	250	238
Trichlorethylene	57	64.5	60	00

A Churchill-Davidson; B Vickers, Morgan & Spencer; C Dunnill & Colvin; D Synopsis

27 Some of the less common medical syndromes have direct relevance to the provision of anaesthesia and may cause difficulties in the use of anaesthetic drugs.

A myasthenia-like syndrome may occur in:
a) hypokalaemia
b) thyrotoxicosis
c) motor neurone disease
d) carcinoma of the thymus
e) bronchogenic carcinoma

28 The muscular dystrophies are an inherited group of conditions whose pathology extends to organ systems other than musculoskeletal.

Common features of dystrophia myotonica include:
a) testicular atrophy
b) cataracts
c) optic atrophy
d) ptosis
e) frontal baldness

References

27.1	Katz & Kadis	p 622–626
27.2	Anaesthesia Review 3	p 20
27.3	OTM	p 22.16–18
27.4	Katz & Kadis	p 615–622
28.1	Katz & Kadis	p 596–600
28.2	Anaesthesia Review 3	p 18
28.3	OTM	p 22.11–12

27 There are many conditions and syndromes which cause myasthenia. The myasthenic syndrome (also called Eaton–Lambert syndrome) is one. They are all characterized by muscle weakness unrelated to nerve traffic. Some have remediable causes, others do not. All cause problems for the anaesthetist either from atypical responses to opioids, barbiturates or muscle relaxants, or from ventilatory and cardiac problems.

a) T The syndromes of familial periodic paralysis, especially the hypokalaemic variety, may present with asymmetric muscle weakness. The pathology does not seem to relate to the neuromuscular junction but rather to the muscle itself (27.1, 27.2, 27.3).

b) T There is a subgroup of the periodic paralyses which responds to thyroidectomy, called 'thyrotoxic periodic paralysis'. There is also a 5% incidence of myasthenia gravis in patients with thyrotoxicosis, which responds to control of thyroid function (27.1, 27.3).

c) F Motor neurone disease shows the features of denervation rather than weakness of the muscle itself (27.3).

d) T Myasthenia gravis may or may not respond to thymectomy. Curiously, those found to have a thymoma at operation tend to progress less well than those who are tumour free (27.1, 27.3, 27.4).

e) T A classical feature of the Eaton–Lambert type of myasthenia syndrome, the tumour only revealing itself long after the syndrome has appeared, though not uncommonly the patient known to have a tumour will develop the syndrome (27.1, 27.3, 27.4).

28 Dystrophia myotonica is one of the multitude of muscular dystrophies. The muscles fail to relax after contraction. Muscle relaxants have unpredictable effects (especially depolarizing agents). Muscle may not relax completely after a depolarizing drug, yet fail to return to appropriate activity when the effect of the drug wears off (28.1).

a) T Testicular atrophy is one of the short string of classical features characterizing dystrophia myotonica (28.1, 28.2, 28.3).

b) T Cataracts are a cardinal feature, said to occur also in generations previous to that of the patient (28.1, 28.2, 28.3).

c) F Optic atrophy is not commonly encountered in dystrophia myotonica, although poor eyesight may be a symptom (28.3).

d) T Ptosis is common in dystrophia myotonica (28.3).

e) T Frontal balding is a well known feature of the disease (28.1, 28.3).

29 Surgery falls within the scope of the Part 3 FRCAnaes examination, to the embarrassment of the less well prepared candidate.

Acute pancreatitis may cause:
a) retroperitoneal abscess
b) pancreatic abscess
c) pancreatic pseudocyst
d) hyperglycaemia
e) tetany

30 Patients with inflammatory bowel diseases may present for frequent and recurrent surgery whilst receiving polypharmacy.

Complications of Crohn's disease include:
a) entero-enteric fistulae
b) bowel perforation
c) recurrence after resection
d) fistula-in-ano
e) lymphoma

References

29.1	Katz & Kadis	p 475–476
29.2	OTM	p 12.183–188
30.1	Katz & Kadis	p 467–468
30.2	OTM	p 12.121–126
30.3	Muir	p 19.33–35

29a) T In that the pancreas is basically a retroperitoneal organ, an abscess can develop (29.1, 29.2).
  b) T In severe acute pancreatitis, the whole of the organ can become necrotic and secondarily infected (29.1, 29.2).
  c) T A pseudocyst is not lined with epithelium as a true cyst would be. Pseudocysts occur commonly and may need to be drained, usually into the stomach (29.1, 29.2).
  d) T Hyperglycaemia occurs from disruption or destruction of the pancreatic islets. This can occur in the acute situation but is more common in chronic pancreatitis or after repeated acute episodes (29.1)
  e) T Calcium may be sequestrated in areas of fat necrosis in the pancreas, leading to a major fall in the circulating concentration of both ionized and unionized calcium. Carpopedal spasm (tetany) may occur (29.1, 29.2).

30a) T Entero-enteric fistulae are frequently seen and may be the presenting problem in Crohn's disease (30.1, 30.2).
  b) T Perforation of the bowel may occur (30.1, 30.2).
  c) T Recurrence after surgery is a classical feature of the disease (30.1, 30.2).
  d) T Fistula-in-ano may complicate Crohn's disease (30.2).
  e) F Although Crohn's disease may be associated with bowel malignancies, especially colonic, lymphomatous association is not usual (30.3).

31 Do not confuse the characteristics of an ideal gas with those of an ideal anaesthetic agent. The question below concerns basic physics only.

The following are true of an ideal gas:
a) the volume of a given mass of gas at a given pressure is inversely proportional to its temperature
b) at constant temperature, the volume of a given mass of gas is directly proportional to its pressure
c) at absolute zero, the volume of a gas would be one volume percent
d) at a given temperature and pressure, one mole of any gas occupies the same volume as one mole of any other gas
e) the Ideal Gas Law is a combination of Boyle's, Charles' and Avogadro's Laws

32 Maximum safe doses of local anaesthetic agents should be second nature. In a viva, this topic will often lead to questioning on the clinical features of toxicity and their treatment.

The following are the recommended maximum doses for local anaesthetic drugs:
a) lignocaine 7 mg/kg
b) bupivacaine 2 mg/kg
c) prilocaine 6 mg/kg
d) bupivacaine with adrenaline 4 mg/kg
e) lignocaine with adrenaline 9 mg/kg

References	
31.1 Ward	p 6
31.2 Parbrook	p 53–56
32.1 Eriksson	p 13
32.2 Dunnill & Colvin	p 19
32.3 Synopsis	p 593–605
32.4 Churchill-Davidson	p 845
32.5 Aitkenhead & Smith	p 459

31a) F This is Charles' law. If the pressure is kept constant and the gas is heated, it will expand by 1/273rd of the original volume for every °C rise in temperature (31.1).
  b) F This is Boyle's law.(This is not the Boyle who invented the anaesthetic machine but the 18th century Boyle.) Boyle's law basically states that at constant temperature, PV = a constant, or to put it another way, P = k/V, i.e. pressure and volume are <u>inversely</u> related (31.1).
  c) F There is no such thing as a real gas at absolute zero (−273 °C). All of the real gases have liquefied long before this, but the concept of an ideal gas is attractive as a physical theory. In this theory, following the gas laws, the volume of a gas will reduce by 1/273rd for every °C fall. This ends up in the slightly ridiculous idea that at absolute zero, the gas has zero volume.
  d) T This is Avogadro's hypothesis and it is borne out by experimentation (31.2).
  e) T (31.2).

32 Minor variations exist between sources. The problem lies in the definition of a toxic dose. It is usually defined in terms of intravenous injection rather than the less predictable but more likely routes of administration. The definition needs to be interpreted carefully. Churchill-Davidson (32.5) quotes maximum doses in terms of epidural bolus, a more likely scenario but with less predictable absorption than the intravenous route, while Eriksson (32.1) refers to maximum dose to a male adult. Refer to Table 3 (32.1, 32.2, 32.3, 32.4, 32.5).
  a) F
  b) T
  c) T
  d) F
  e) F

Table 3 Maximum doses of local anaesthetics from various sources (mg/kg)

Source	A	B	C	D
Lignocaine	2–3	3	3	5
Bupivacaine	2	2	2	2
Prilocaine	6	6	4	6
Bupivacaine + adrenaline	–	2	2	–
Lignocaine + adrenaline	–	7	7	–

A Dunnill & Colvin; B Eriksson; C Synopsis; D Aitkenhead & Smith

33 Methaemoglobinaemia is a source of diagnostic confusion in clinical practice because of the apparent cyanosis. If there is significant methaemoglobinaemia then there will be an equivalent reduction in oxygen transport.

Methaemoglobinaemia may be caused by:
a) the treatment of cyanide poisoning
b) lignocaine
c) prilocaine
d) a congenital condition
e) glyceryl trinitrate

34 The physics and behaviour of water and its vapour play a large part in respiratory physiology. Humidifiers often appear in written, MCQ and viva formats, and questions are often related to the physical principles of vaporization.

Humidity:
a) expressed in absolute units, relates the amount of water present to the maximum amount possible at that temperature
b) expressed in absolute units, is the mass of water in unit volume of gas at ambient pressure and temperature
c) is a measure of the total water content in the gas, both vapour and droplets
d) expressed in relative units, compares the humidity at ambient temperature to that at absolute zero
e) in the lungs is usually 95–100% of the maximum possible

References

33.1	Vickers, Morgan & Spencer	p 346
33.2	Churchill-Davidson	p 185
33.3	Synopsis	p 601
33.4	BMJ (1991) 303	p 695
34.1	Ward	p 242
34.2	Ganong	p 599

33 Normal haemoglobin contains iron in the ferrous form. Oxidation of this iron to the ferric form causes an increase in the affinity of the molecule for oxygen and, if this is widespread, a reduced oxygen availability to the tissues. The oxidized molecule is methaemoglobin, of which there is always a small amount present in the circulation, but at low concentrations it will not present a problem. Although recognition of methaemoglobin as the cause of cyanosis may be difficult, the treatment should be straightforward. Methylene blue is given by injection, or vitamin C by mouth; both act as reducing agents.

a) **T** One of the standard treatments of cyanide poisoning is the formation of cyan-methaemoglobin by the administration of sodium nitrite, to combine with the cyanide ion. Cyan-methaemoglobin then dissociates into methaemoglobin and cyanide, which is converted to thiocyanate by using sodium thiosulphate (33.1).

b) **T** Surprising but true (33.3, 33.4).

c) **T** The dose needed to cause significant methaemoglobinaemia is large; in excess of 900 mg – over twice the recommended maximum (33.1, 33.2, 33.3, 32.1).

d) **T** Some people have the misfortune to have a congenitally higher concentration of methaemoglobin than normal. They are treated with high doses of vitamin C as a reducing agent (33.1, 33.2).

e) **T** All of the organic nitrites and nitrates can cause methaemoglobinaemia if given in sufficient quantity (33.1 33.2).

34a) **F** This is the definition of relative humidity, it looks at one situation relative to the maximum possible at the same temperature and pressure (34.1).

b) **T** This is the definition of absolute humidity (34.1).

c) **F** Not droplets, only vapour. The presence of droplets would suggest that the vapour was supersaturated and therefore the relative humidity would be greater than 100% (34.1).

d) **F** The two are compared at the same temperature and pressure (34.1).

e) **T** Passage of dry gas through the nasal passages and the trachea will saturate the gas with water, reaching a partial pressure of 47 mmHg, the saturated vapour pressure of water at 37°C which is the maximum attainable (34.2).

35 All anaesthetists should be able to recognize and treat the more common or more important forms of drug toxicity. Often, general principles of resuscitation and support are all that is necessary but there are some specific treatments for specific poisons.

In the treatment of poisoning, the following could be used:
a) atropine in paracetamol poisoning
b) physostigmine in imipramine poisoning
c) intermittent positive pressure ventilation in salicylate poisoning
d) methionine in paraquat poisoning
e) dicobalt edetate in cyanide poisoning

36 Take extreme care with this question; read it very carefully and study the wording.

The following would lead you to doubt the diagnosis of acute appendicitis in a five-year-old boy:
a) temperature 40°C
b) pain in the right iliac fossa when pressing on the left side
c) diarrhoea on the evening before admission
d) proteinuria
e) productive cough

References		
35.1	Goodman & Gilman	p 658–659
35.2	OTM	p 6.18–20
35.3	Goodman & Gilman	p 411–413
35.4	Goodman & Gilman	p 651–652
35.5	Goodman & Gilman	p 1654
35.6	OTM	p 6.11–12
35.7	OTM	p 6.56
36.1	Giles	p 1161–1163

35a) F The treatment of paracetamol poisoning includes gastric lavage, administration of activated charcoal followed by methionine or N-acetyl cysteine followed by salt and protein restriction to relieve the load upon the failing liver. Anticholinergic agents are not indicated (35.1, 35.2).

b) T Poisoning with tricyclic antidepressants can produce varied signs including excitation, restlessness, convulsions, respiratory depression, coma and hypotension, as well as the more commonly seen tachyarrhythmias. Physostigmine has been used to counter the antimuscarinic cardiac and neurological effects of tricyclic poisoning because of its ability to cross the blood–brain barrier (35.3).

c) T The early signs of salicylate poisoning include hyperventilation. This is replaced later by respiratory depression and coma, which may require respiratory support (35.4).

d) F Paraquat is a herbicide which is notorious for its toxic effects if not handled correctly. Indeed, it has been used as an agent in chemical warfare. The results of poisoning with this chemical are: pulmonary oedema leading to fibrosis, and renal failure. There seems to be no place for methionine in the treatment of poisoning with this agent. There seems to be little that can be done except supportive measures, however haemodialysis has been advocated (35.5, 35.6).

e) T Dicobalt edetate forms stable compounds with cyanide, thus protecting the haemoglobin molecule. This has become the standard treatment for cyanide poisoning, rather than the use of sodium nitrite and thiosulphate as previously. The diagnosis should be secure because the dicobalt edetate is itself toxic (35.7).

36 Appendicitis is one of the most common abdominal emergencies. The incidence of incorrect diagnosis prior to appendicectomy is of the order of 20% (36.1). Remember that the question said 'would lead you to doubt', not 'these are the features of'.

a) T Although most children with appendicitis have a fever, it is not usually so high. This degree of pyrexia would suggest a viral illness (36.1).

b) T Pressure in the left iliac fossa causing pain in the right iliac fossa does not fit the usual picture of guarding and tenderness in the right iliac fossa but, rather, suggests a viral cause, perhaps mesenteric adenitis (36.1).

c) T Diarrhoea may suggest a cause other than appendicitis (36.1).

d) F Proteinuria is quite common in acute appendicitis (36.1).

e) T Acute chest infections occasionally mimic appendicitis, probably because of the generalized lymphadenopathy which accompanies the illness.

37 Surgery is indicated in the following:
  a) single thyroid nodule
  b) papillary carcinoma of the thyroid
  c) thyrotoxicosis
  d) retrosternal goitre
  e) Hashimoto's thyroiditis

38 Clinical questions can prove difficult as there will always be some room for debate. Multiple choice examinations are marked by their lack of opportunity for such debate.

A previously fit young man presents to the Accident and Emergency Department. He is cyanosed, breathless and his trachea is deviated to the left. He needs:
  a) measurement of arterial blood gas tensions before any therapy is carried out
  b) supplementary oxygen administration
  c) urgent chest X-ray
  d) immediate needling of the right side of his chest
  e) an electrocardiogram

References

37.1 Giles   p 864–871

38.1 Shoemaker   p 1246
38.2 Kaplan   p 467–472

37 This is is an ambiguous question in that some of the answers are 'it depends on whether...'. The stem says IS indicated rather than MAY BE.

a) **T** Surgery MAY be indicated for a single nodule, it depends upon the results of investigations such as ultrasound and needling. Is the nodule solid or cystic, is it 'hot' or 'cold'? A cold nodule on radioisotope imaging would be more serious than a hot one (37.1).

b) **T** The lesion can be very widespread within the organ. There are two schools of thought: either that the gland should be removed in total and then investigations carried out to find residual tissue; or that most of the gland should be removed and the rest suppressed by hormonal manipulation. Either way, the patient undergoes surgery (37.1).

c) **F** Thyroidectomy is not the first-line treatment it was some years ago. Medical treatment is the first line, and surgery reserved for medical failures or for large goitres and those causing pressure symptoms (37.1).

d) **F** But it depends upon the symptoms. If the patient is having symptoms of superior mediastinal syndrome or of tracheal compression then surgery is indicated, otherwise not (37.1).

e) **F** Hashimoto's autoimmune thyroiditis may produce a large goitre in the early stages of the disease, but this is self-limiting and the thyroid eventually shrinks away to nothing (37.1).

38 This question defies references. One is led to assume that the patient has a right-sided tension pneumothorax. The information left out is important. Has he any difference in the percussion of the two sides of the chest? What was he doing at the time? What are his pulse and blood pressure? Has he got a knife sticking out of his chest? Is he very tall with long fingers and a high arch to his palate? Let us assume that this unfortunate has a right-sided tension pneumothorax, but haemothorax is another possibility. (38.1, 38.2).

a) **F** If he is cyanosed he will have a low Pa_{O_2}

b) **T** Good idea! Not that he will be able to make much use of it.

c) **F** By the time the machine has arrived or the patient has been moved to the radiology department it will be too late.

d) **T** Any type of needle will do, as long as it is inserted above rather than below a rib and in the mid-thorax in the mid-axillary line. This manoeuvre will confirm or refute the diagnosis: no air, no pneumothorax.

e) **F** An electrocardiogram will not supply useful information for the acute management of the patient.

39 The Valsalva manoeuvre can be used in the diagnosis of a number of medical and physiological conditions. The manoeuvre itself is not necessarily the formal affair of blowing against a mercury column, but includes any kind of straining against a closed glottis.

At the end of the Valsalva manoeuvre, there is no fall in heart rate if there is:
a) cervical spondylosis
b) left-sided heart failure
c) autonomic neuropathy
d) Horner's syndrome
e) aortic valve regurgitation

40 Complications and unwanted effects of drugs are very frequent topics. It is wise to be careful of minutiae. Be very sure of your facts on a particular drug before stating that a certain side effect is not seen.

The following drugs may cause enlargement of the thyroid gland:
a) carbimazole
b) lithium
c) nifedipine
d) phenylbutazone
e) omeprazole

References

39.1	OTM	p 21.77–78
39.2	Davidson	p 297
39.3	Gray	p 803
40.1	Vickers, Morgan & Spencer	p 434
40.2	Data Sheet Compendium	p 425
40.3	Data Sheet Compendium	p 128
40.4	Data Sheet Compendium	p 558
40.5	Goodman & Gilman	p 902–904

39 The Valsalva manoeuvre involves increasing the intrathoracic pressure suddenly to 30–40 mmHg and maintaining this pressure for several seconds before release. Changes in heart rate are dependent upon intact baroreceptor reflexes, autonomic nervous activity and normal brain-stem traffic (39.1).

  a) F Cervical spondylosis, being a bone and joint disease, would seem to have no connection with this manoeuvre. However, ankylosing spondylitis is associated with aortic regurgitation, although this should make no difference to the answer (see **e**) (39.2).

  b) T In left heart failure there is both an increased intrathoracic blood volume and a failure of the ventricle to compensate for changes in filling pressure. There will be no compensating changes in rate or pressure at the end of the manoeuvre (39.1).

  c) T The failure of the autonomic nervous system, as in diabetes or the Shy–Drager syndrome, will mean that there is no peripheral vaso-constriction and no autonomic change in heart rate at any time during the test (39.1).

  d) T Horner's syndrome is the result of a block, from whatever cause, of the stellate ganglion. This sympathetic ganglion is formed from the inferior cervical and the first thoracic ganglia. Among the many branches of the stellate ganglion are the middle and inferior cardiac nerves, which form the cardiac plexus of sympathetic nerves around the heart and great vessels. This plexus, along with the vagus, controls the cardiac rate. If the stellate ganglion is blocked, causing a Horner's syndrome, then the changes in rate at the end of the Valsalva manoeuvre cannot happen (39.1, 39.3).

  e) F Aortic regurgitation should only exaggerate the effects of the test. In the initial phase of increased pressure there will not be such a great increase in blood pressure. Because the increase in pressure raises cardiac afterload, the regurgitation will increase, blood pressure will fall further and heart rate will increase more as the peripheral circulation compensates. At the release point there will be a great increase in cardiac output as the afterload falls and an even greater fall in heart rate than usual.

40a) T (40.1).
  b) T (40.2).
  c) F (40.3).
  d) T (40.4).
  e) F (40.5).

41 **In clinical practice at sea level, the saturated vapour pressure of all commonly used anaesthetic vapours and gases:**
 a) equals their boiling point
 b) equals atmospheric pressure at their boiling point
 c) is the highest partial pressure of the vapour that can be achieved under the prevailing physical conditions
 d) varies with the barometric pressure
 e) varies with temperature

42 Surgical biochemistry provides the basis for this question. There is useful information in the stem.

 A 48-year-old woman has undergone elective cholecystectomy. 36 hours postoperatively she becomes oliguric with a blood urea 30 mmol/l, (preoperative value 10 mmol/l). The urine osmolality is 290 mosmol/kg. The following statements are true:
 a) the preoperative urea concentration excludes acute renal failure as a diagnosis
 b) the patient is dehydrated
 c) the urine osmolality suggests acute renal failure
 d) a fluid challenge of two litres of lactated Ringer's solution (Hartmann's solution) should be given
 e) diuretics are contraindicated

References

41.1	Parbrook	p 76
41.2	Parbrook	p 148
42.1	Whitby, Smith & Beckett	p 150–173
42.2	Dunnill & Colvin	p 139

41 The saturated vapour pressure (SVP) of a gas or vapour is a physical constant for that agent. It varies with ambient temperature but not pressure. SVP is the highest vapour pressure that can be achieved under the prevailing conditions. When SVP equals atmospheric pressure, the liquid boils; the temperature at which this occurs is the boiling point and this varies with pressure. For example: the SVP of water at 37°C is 47 mmHg, the boiling point of water at sea level is 100°C. The SVP at 100°C is 760 mmHg. If the ambient pressure is lowered, the temperature at which the SVP equals ambient pressure will also be lower. Hence, high-level mountaineers use pressure cookers to bring the pressure back up to 760 mmHg and the boiling point to 100°C. Note that the stem of this question states 'at sea level', i.e. under normal atmospheric pressure (41.1, 41.2).

a) F A nonsense statement. How can a pressure equal a temperature?
b) T See the explanation above.
c) T But SVP could be increased by increasing the temperature.
d) F Although SVP varies with temperature. Do not confuse the two.
e) T As described above.

42 The question assumes a knowledge of the normal ranges for blood urea and osmolality and the normal range for urine osmolality. The fact that this 48-year-old has a raised urea preoperatively (normal is up to 6.5 mmol/l depending on laboratory) suggests some pre-existing renal dysfunction which may be exacerbated by the fluid stresses of surgery. The rise to 30 mmol/l postoperatively is greater than would be expected due to the catabolic response to surgery alone. While this might be a result of pre-renal factors such as dehydration, the only other result available suggests otherwise. If the serum sodium concentration or the CVP were quoted there might be some support for dehydration, but the fact that the quoted urine osmolality is the same as the normal for blood (250–295 mosm/l) suggests that the urine is glomerular filtrate and that there is acute tubular dysfunction if not necrosis (42.1, 42.2).

a) F The preoperative result is abnormal but in isolation will not indicate the subsequent course of events.
b) F Bald statements such as this are usually false unless supported by significant evidence. This one is not.
c) T The normal range for urine osmolality is variously quoted as 300–1000 or 400–1400 mosmol/kg. Either way, this result is low and the urine is not being concentrated by the tubules.
d) F A two-litre fluid challenge is excessive even if the diagnosis were dehydration, which it is not. The correct use of fluid challenges would be 500 ml at a time and preferably under CVP control, but not in the face of acute tubular dysfunction.
e) T Incremental doses of frusemide may help in the diagnosis and help to re-establish urine flow. This is the standard initial treatment for this condition. In the past much larger doses were used – 500 mg at a time – which were shown to be pointless.

43 Patients suffering from diabetes mellitus are met frequently in everyday practice. Questions on the disease process will not always have direct relevance to choice of anaesthetic technique.

In diabetes mellitus:
a) corneal opacification is common
b) retinopathy occurs early
c) ketonuria is a common presentation of the non-insulin dependent type
d) may result in painful ulcers of the feet
e) serial glucose tolerance tests may be useful in monitoring control

44 A raised arterial P_{CO_2} is found in:
a) those acclimatized to high altitude
b) the 'Pickwickian' syndrome
c) early septic shock
d) acidosis from renal causes
e) infusion of bicarbonate

References

43.1	OTM	p 9.82–86
43.2	OTM	p 9.56
43.3	OTM	p 9.76–78
44.1	Nunn	p 312–317
44.2	Stoelting	p 545
44.3	Guyton	p 444–450
44.4	Tinker	p 265
44.5	Davidson	p 585

43a) F Diabetic eye disease is one of the main causes of blindness in the UK. It usually takes the form of retinopathy and, less commonly, cataract. Corneal opacity is not often a feature of diabetes (43.1).

b) F Diabetic retinopathy is common but not an early feature. Only 4% of diabetics have retinopathy at diagnosis. It commonly develops some 10–20 years after diagnosis (43.1).

c) F Ketonuria is a frequent feature of the presentation of the insulin dependent type of diabetes, not the non-insulin dependent type. Non-insulin dependent diabetics only tend to become ketotic if they suffer a severe illness (43.2).

d) F The leg and foot ulcers which develop in diabetes are painless rather than painful, because of the neuropathy which is commonly found in these patients (43.1).

e) F The glucose tolerance test is used in the diagnosis rather than the control of diabetics. Short term control is assessed with blood and urine glucose measurements, while long term control is monitored by fructosamine and HbA1 measurements (43.3).

44a) F Acclimatization to high altitude involves marked hyperventilation due to the hypoxic drive to ventilation in the presence of a low partial pressure of oxygen. The arterial P_{CO_2} may be as low as 1 kPa (7.5 mmHg). There is a syndrome of chronic mountain sickness in permanent high altitude residents (Monge's syndrome), where the ventilatory response to hypoxia becomes obtunded. The Pa_{O_2} falls and Pa_{CO_2} rises. Cyanosis and pulmonary hypertension are features of this condition (44.1).

b) T Pickwickian syndrome, also known as the sleep apnoea syndrome, is characterized by obesity, lethargy and an elevated Pa_{CO_2}. It is named from the fat boy in Dickens' 'The Pickwick Papers', who was always falling asleep. The Pa_{CO_2} may fall with weight loss (44.2).

c) F In early sepsis there is a rise in temperature and increased neural drive to respiration, before an increase in CO_2 production. These factors increase the minute volume of ventilation, reducing the arterial P_{CO_2} (44.3, 44.4).

d) F The contrary is true. In renal acidotic states, the Pa_{CO_2} tends to fall because of the acidotic stimulus to respiration, which acts to restore the pH by imposing a respiratory alkalosis on the renal acidosis(44.5).

e) T Infusion of bicarbonate (a metabolic alkalosis), will consume hydrogen ions to form carbonic acid which dissociates to CO_2 and water. The fall in hydrogen ion concentration depresses respiration, increasing Pa_{CO_2} and tending to return the pH toward normal by dissociation of dissolved carbonic acid to yield bicarbonate and hydrogen ions. The bicarbonate concentration will therefore stay high in the presence of a high Pa_{CO_2} until the kidneys restore the status quo (44.3).

45 Wheeze is a musical sound which is produced when airway narrowing results in oscillation. Wheeze may be a symptom or a sign.

Wheeze may be caused by:
a) tumour
b) foreign body
c) secretions
d) asthma
e) pulmonary oedema

46 The physiological changes in pregnancy have direct relevance to anaesthesia and are very frequent examination topics.

In pregnancy:
a) plasma fibrinogen concentration increases
b) the increase in cardiac output is by increased stroke volume only
c) the cardiac output increases by about 50% overall
d) the functional residual capacity is reduced
e) the residual volume increases

References

45.1 Souhami & Moxham   p 462

46.1 Moir   p 14
46.2 Moir   p 17–33
46.3 Scurr, Feldman & Soni   p 192
46.4 Report on Confidential Enquiries   p 37–45
       into Maternal Deaths in the United
       Kingdom 1985–1987

45a) T Causes of airway narrowing will produce wheeze. The sound will change according to the cause of the wheeze. Tumour, if causing compression, gives rise to localized wheeze of monophonic note (45.1).
  b) T Localized wheezing will be produced with a similar sound to that caused by tumour as described above (45.1).
  c) T The presence of bronchial secretions causes wheezing (45.1).
  d) T Asthma is the most common cause of wheezing. Usually this will be expiratory, generalized and polyphonic in nature (45.1).
  e) T Generalized wheeze will be heard (45.1).

46a) T The blood of pregnant women is hypercoagulable and there is thus a tendency to spontaneous coagulation, resulting in deep venous thrombosis or pulmonary embolism. Pulmonary embolism is a major cause of maternal death, detailed in the Report on Confidential Enquiries into Maternal Deaths. Fibrinogen concentration rises from 2.5–4 g/l to 5 g/l (46.1, 46.3, 46.4).
  b) F There is a contribution from an increase in heart rate (46.2).
  c) F The increase in cardiac output is about 33% (46.2).
  d) T The FRC falls from about 1620 ml to about 1325 ml (46.2).
  e) F The residual volume falls from about 965 ml to about 770 ml (46.2).

47 Regarding the blood supply of the heart:
a) the right coronary artery runs in the anterior atrio-ventricular groove
b) the coronary sinus is in the anterior atrio-ventricular groove
c) the venae cordi minimi (Thebesian veins) drain directly into the cardiac chambers
d) there are no anastamoses between the right and left coronary circulations
e) the atrio-ventricular node is supplied by the left coronary artery

48 Fat embolism is a major and common complication of orthopaedic surgery and bony trauma which can prove fatal.

Fat embolism may cause:
a) a raised arterial P_{CO_2}
b) oedema of the retina
c) petechial haemorrhages over the upper chest
d) pyrexia
e) hypocalcaemia

References

47.1	Gray	p 729–731
47.2	Gray	p 792–793
47.3	Nunn	p 167
48.1	Nunn	p 449
48.2	Nunn	p 170
48.3	Synopsis	p 788
48.4	Miller	p 1964

47a) T The right coronary artery arises above the right anterior cusp of the aortic valve (usually) and runs downward and to the right in the anterior A-V groove to reach the inferior border of the heart before turning onto the diaphragmatic surface, still in the A-V groove (47.1).

b) F The coronary sinus is the main venous drainage of the heart. It lies in the posterior A-V groove (47.2).

c) T The Thebesian veins drain directly into the cardiac cavities. This explains the origin of some, but not all, of the difference in oxygen partial pressure between blood from the pulmonary veins and the aorta (47.2, 47.3).

d) F There is a remarkable degree of cross-coronary anastamosis demonstrable anatomically, far more than was once thought. This tends to be at the level of small subendocardial vessels rather than main arteries (47.1).

e) F The A-V node is usually supplied by the left coronary artery but may be supplied by the right in about 10–20% of cases (47.1).

48 Fat embolism is a common problem in patients with bony fractures. While it usually presents more than 24 hours after injury, it can occur almost immediately after injury or up to several days later. The effects are mainly cerebral and pulmonary, causing confusion with hypoxia. There may also be a coagulopathy and cardiovascular collapse.

a) F Initially there is an increase in physiological deadspace and later shunting because of pulmonary arterial spasm as a result of the toxic effects of the embolized fat. Hyperventilation is usually present so that even large shunts do not result in elevated arterial P_{CO_2} (48.1, 48.2).

b) F Note that there may be fat globules visible in the retinal arteries (48.3).

c) T Petechiae are one of the cardinal signs of fat embolism (48.4). Their absence does not refute the diagnosis, however.

d) T The pyrexia is related to the fat embolus, not to the injury which precedes it (48.3).

e) T Hypocalcaemia may vary in magnitude (48.3).

49 The effects and management of decompression sickness ('the bends') are important, not only because of the need for immediate specialized treatment but also because of the physical and physiological principles illustrated.

Decompression sickness:
a) may have a delayed onset
b) may lead to aseptic necrosis of the femoral head
c) may cause paralysis
d) can be treated with a helium–oxygen mixture
e) is due to changes in the alveolar–arterial oxygen gradient

50 Methyldopa may cause:
a) haemolytic anaemia
b) increased sensitivity to inhalational anaesthetic agents
c) positive direct Coombs test
d) interference with diagnostic tests for phaeochromocytoma
e) toxic hepatitis

References

49.1 Churchill-Davidson	p 150–154
49.2 Shoemaker	p 526–529
49.3 Guyton	p 473–474
50.1 Goodman & Gilman	p 791
50.2 Miller	p 1798
50.3 Data Sheet Compendium	p 1041

49 Decompression sickness seems at first sight to be obscure. It need not be. Diving below five metres is quite common for sporting divers breathing air. Professional divers need not necessarily be North Sea oil rig saturation divers. Any tunnelling activity where increased ambient pressure is used to exclude water may lead to decompression sickness.

a) T This depends on the definition of 'delayed onset'. Some of the results of decompression sickness may only become apparent in the long term. Bone necrosis is one of them (vide infra). It is said that any diver who has been below five metres should not fly, even in a pressurized aircraft, within 24 hours of diving because he will still be supersaturated with nitrogen during this time (49.1, 49.3).

b) T Aseptic necrosis of the femoral head is the best known long-term complication of decompression sickness. It results from multiple decompressions over a long period of time, as in a professional diver (49.1).

c) T The blood supply to the spinal cord is precarious at the best of times. The bubbles of nitrogen formed during too rapid decompression may occlude the small spinal arteries, causing paralysis (49.1).

d) F Treatment is usually by recompression with either air or oxygen, depending on the pressure needed. Oxygen alone cannot be used at greater than two atmospheres because of high-pressure toxicity and pulmonary oxygen toxicity. Remember that saturation diving does indeed take place in a helium–oxygen environment, but this is far from the only mixture which may be used (49.1).

e) F The problem in decompression sickness is that the patient is supersaturated with nitrogen when at depth and has decompressed in such a way that the nitrogen dissolved in the tissues is released at a rate faster than the circulation and lungs can eliminate it. The partial pressure of nitrogen exceeds the solubility coefficient, which causes bubbles to appear in the tissues and circulation, with results according to the site of the bubble (49.1, 49.2).

50a) T Haemolytic anaemia is the best remembered side effect of the drug. It is seen in about 5% of those patients who have been receiving methyldopa for at least six months (50.1).

b) T There appears to be no logical explanation for this phenomenon. The minimum alveolar concentration (MAC) of the inhalational agents is reduced in patients receiving methyldopa (50.2).

c) T Coomb's positivity is a feature of the haemolytic anaemia and is one of the better remembered side effects (50.1).

d) T Methyldopa fluoresces at the same wavelengths of light as the catecholamines. Therefore, in urine tests for catecholamines which rely on fluoroscopy there will be a falsely elevated result and a false positive diagnosis. Tests which rely upon the conversion of vanillyl-mandelic acid (VMA) to vanillin will not be affected (50.3).

e) T Some patients taking methyldopa develop liver enzymatic changes which mimic infective hepatitis. Liver function tests return to normal on withdrawal of the drug (50.1).

51 Phaeochromocytoma is an adrenal tumour which is derived from chromaffin cells. Extra-adrenal chromaffin tumours are known as paragangliomata.

The following conditions are associated with phaeochromocytoma:
a) bronchiectasis
b) medullary carcinoma of the thyroid gland
c) primary hyperaldosteronism
d) tuberous sclerosis
e) neurofibromatosis

52 Contraindications to surgery can provide an interesting perspective on pathological lesions. They seem to be dwindling!

Surgery for carcinoma of the bronchus is usually contraindicated by:
a) atrial fibrillation
b) peripheral neuropathy
c) superior mediastinal syndrome
d) empyema
e) left recurrent laryngeal nerve palsy

References		
51.1	Muir	p 26.40
51.2	Stoelting	p 502
51.3	Katz & Kadis	p 276–279
52.1	Churchill-Davidson	p 740
52.2	Trends	p 149
52.3	Souhami & Moxham	p 534

51a) F There is no described connection between phaeochromocytoma and bronchiectasis.

b) T Multiple adenomas and adenocarcinomas may occur together (51.1, 51.2, 51.3).

c) F Phaeochromocytoma is a condition of catecholamine-secreting tissue: adrenal medulla and postganglionic sympathetic fibres. Primary hyperaldosteronism is a condition of the adrenal cortex, usually unilateral because of tumour but occasionally bilateral due to adrenal hyperplasia. The two are thus problems of different organs (51.2).

d) T Tuberous sclerosis is a condition characterized by epilepsy, mental deficiency and adenoma sebaceum. There is a definite association between this condition, phaeochromocytoma and neurofibromatosis (51.2, 51.3).

e) T As described above (51.1, 51.2, 51.3).

52 Who decides what is a contraindication to surgery? One man's contraindication is another man's minor problem. 'Surgery for carcinoma of the bronchus' could apply to one of several types of lobectomy or a pneumonectomy.

a) F Although controlled rhythms other than sinus, and especially those involving ventricular abnormalities, carry a major increase in the risk of thoracic surgery, atrial fibrillation itself is not a contraindication unless it is associated with congestive failure, in which case the extra pulmonary vascular resistance after a pneumonectomy could be embarrassing to the point of death (52.1).

b) F There is a condition known as carcinomatous neuropathy where motor weakness is out of proportion to the advance of a bronchial tumour. It is characterized by demyelination and atrophy of muscle fibres. This does not appear to be related to the myasthenic (Eaton–Lambert) syndrome (52.1). The response given here is the authors' choice.

c) T The superior mediastinal syndrome is the result of obstruction of the superior vena cava, usually by tumour compression within the upper lobes. Treatment is palliative, although venous bypass procedures are possible (52.2).

d) T Empyema, an infected pleural effusion, must be a contraindication to any open chest procedure until it is drained or dry. It may be an indication of transpleural spread (52.3).

e) T The left recurrent laryngeal nerve follows a course under the arch of the aorta at the point where the ligamentum arteriosum is attached. This area also contains the lymph nodes which drain the bronchi. Therefore, a recurrent laryngeal palsy may suggest that a bronchial tumour on that side has already metastasized and may not be operable.

53 Patterns of tumour metastasis are variable. There are, however, some common associations.

The following tumours commonly metastasize to bone:
a) adenocarcinoma of the large intestine
b) bronchial carcinoma
c) papillary carcinoma of the thyroid
d) nephroblastoma (Wilms' tumour)
e) adenocarcinoma of the prostate

54 Because of an active immunization policy, severe tetanus is uncommon in this country, but it may still be encountered from time to time.

Tetanus:
a) is caused by an aerobic organism
b) often occurs with no history of trauma
c) confers immunity for future episodes
d) is satisfactorily treated by tetanus immunoglobulin alone
e) causes autonomic overactivity

References

53.1	Muir	p 19.65–67
53.2	Muir	p 16.65–72
53.3	Muir	p 26.25
53.4	Muir	p 22.63
53.5	Muir	p 25.7–11
54.1	Stoelting	p 652–653
54.2	Churchill-Davidson	p 338–340
54.3	Katz & Kadis	p 717

53a) F Spread of intestinal adenocarcinoma is usually by direct extension or lymphatic spread rather than blood-borne or to bone (53.1).

b) T While direct or lymphatic spread is common, bony metastasis is also seen frequently, especially to vertebrae (53.2).

c) F Papillary thyroid tumours rarely metastasize to bone (53.3).

d) F Wilms' tumour tends to spread directly and to grow along the renal vein to the inferior vena cava rather than to bone (53.4).

e) T Adenocarcinoma of the prostate is notorious for its frequent and widespread bony metastases, especially vertebral and pelvic. Metastases may present before the primary lesion (53.5).

54 Tetanus is a big problem around the world, killing thousands every year. It is much less of a problem in the UK.

a) F The tetanus bacillus (*Clostridium tetani*) is an <u>an</u>aerobic Gram-positive spore-forming rod (54.1, 54.2).

b) T In the UK, there has usually been trauma but it may have been too insignificant for the patient to seek attention. In other countries, the bacilli may have entered through other portals, such as the umbilicus in babies (54.2).

c) F A clinical episode of tetanus does not confer immunity for the future; a full course of immunization is necessary. The usual immunization schedule will not confer permanent immunity and needs 'booster' doses (54.2).

d) F Following trauma which is likely to lead to tetanus, the immunoglobulin may prevent the onset of clinical tetanus. During a clinical episode, the immunoglobulin will only combat the tetanospasmin toxin which is in the periphery rather than in the nervous system. Further tetanospasmin will be produced by bacilli remaining in the wound unless it is debrided and antibiotics given. Time alone will treat the toxin which is within the nervous system, though intrathecal immunoglobulin has been tried. An appropriate system of increasing sedation and ventilatory support according to the degree of spasm and paralysis must also be instituted (54.2).

e) T Even with heavily sedated and paralysed patients there can be frequent and life-threatening autonomic 'storms' consisting of labile hypertension, brady- and tachyarrythmias, hyperpyrexia and other sympathetic effects (54.1, 54.2, 54.3).

55 A thorough grounding in clinical medicine will prove invaluable in revising for the Part 3 FRCAnaes. Diagnosis and management of incidental conditions is part of anaesthetic management.

Cushing's syndrome may show the following features:
a) hypernatraemia
b) hypokalaemia
c) postural hypotension
d) osteoporosis
e) hypercalcaemia

56 **Reflex pulmonary vasoconstriction may be abolished by:**
a) hypoxia
b) tolazoline
c) adrenaline
d) nitrous oxide
e) hypocapnia

References

55.1	Stoelting	p 493–495
55.2	Miller	p 804
56.1	Nunn	p 127–130
56.2	Goodman & Gilman	p 225–226
56.3	Kaplan	p 207–211
56.4	Recent Advances 16	p 20

55a) T Sodium retention and potassium loss are hallmarks of glucocorticoid excess. Despite fluid retention there will be both hypernatraemia and hypokalaemia (55.1).

b) T As described above (55.1).

c) F Patients suffering from Cushing's syndrome are usually hypertensive rather than hypotensive and have increased circulating plasma volume (55.1).

d) T Osteoporosis is one of the classical features of Cushing's syndrome whether it is naturally occurring or iatrogenic. There is a significant loss of bone protein and a failure of calcium absorption (55.1, 55.2).

e) F In Cushing's syndrome there is a failure of calcium absorption. Miller (55.2) comments that the glucocorticoids also have mineralocorticoid activity and so patients with Cushing's syndrome will also show some of the features of Conn's syndrome. This effect can cause tetany because of low serum calcium concentrations.

56 Reflex (also known as hypoxic) pulmonary vasoconstriction may divert blood flow away from poorly ventilated areas of lung and towards better ventilated areas, reducing the effects of ventilation–perfusion mismatch. The relation between pulmonary vasoconstriction and pulmonary hypertension is an inverse one. Vasoconstriction can be reduced by increases in pulmonary blood flow and pressure. This feature is a peculiarity of the resistance of pulmonary vessels (56.1). The pulmonary circulation tends to behave in the opposite way to the systemic circulation where responses to vasoactive substances are concerned.

a) F Which is why it is also known as hypoxic pulmonary vasoconstriction (56.1).

b) T The alpha blocking drugs reduce pulmonary hypoxic vasoconstriction (56.2).

c) F The effects of adrenaline depend to some extent on which receptor predominates in the tissue under consideration. Adrenaline has no vasodilator effect on pulmonary vasculature (56.1).

d) F Nitrous oxide usually has a slight pulmonary vasodilator effect but in pulmonary hypertension causes increases in both pulmonary vascular resistance and pressure (56.3, 56.4).

e) T A fall in Pa_{CO_2} causes a rise in pulmonary artery pressure and therefore a reduction in hypoxic vasoconstriction. Similarly, hypercapnia has a pulmonary vasoconstrictor effect (56.1, 56.3).

57 Pregnancy is not without its problems, which may include disseminated intravascular coagulation. Refer also to question 46.

Disseminated intravascular coagulation (DIC) in pregnancy:
a) may be a sign of amniotic fluid embolism
b) may occur in the presence of a normal platelet count
c) may complicate septicaemia
d) is a late sign in pre-eclampsia
e) plasma fibrinogen degradation products (FDPs) must be greater than 10 μg/l to be diagnostic

58 The anatomy of the epidural space has direct practical relevance. The boundaries and contents of the space feature frequently in examinations. Be prepared to draw a diagram.

The epidural space:
a) is a closed space
b) lies between the spinal dura mater and the arachnoid mater
c) continues through the foramen magnum into the skull
d) ends at about the second sacral segment
e) contains veins whose valves direct flow into the azygos system

References

57.1	Moir	p 288
57.2	Moir	p 281
57.3	Report on Confidential Enquiries into Maternal Deaths 1985–1987	
57.4	Scurr, Feldman & Soni	p 177
57.5	de Gruchy	p 442–445
57.6	Scurr, Feldman & Soni	p 194–195
57.7	Scurr, Feldman & Soni	p 200
58.1	Scurr, Feldman & Soni	p 22–30
58.2	Macintosh	p 53–54

57a) T Amniotic fluid embolism is one of those extremely rare conditions which are difficult to treat because they are so rare that no-one is familiar (by exposure) with the management. The general features are those of a syndrome similar to fat embolism. Predisposing factors include strong uterine contractions, uterine trauma, premature placental separation, uterine stimulation and multiparity. Mortality is around 80%! The clinical signs and symptoms are sudden onset of respiratory distress with cyanosis and a bleeding tendency (57.1, 57.2, 57.3, 57.4).

b) T There are two varieties of DIC; acute and chronic. The chronic form follows intra-uterine fetal death and pre-eclampsia, whereas the acute form is the result of placental abruption, amniotic embolus or similar acute causes. In the chronic form, the clotting factors and the platelet count may be normal because they are being replaced as they are consumed, whereas the bleeding time and FDPs may be altered (57.3).

c) T DIC in pregnancy can be triggered by sepsis, especially in the uterus and genital tract. Septicaemia of any origin is one of the several causes of coagulopathy (57.3, 57.5).

d) T Regular monitoring of coagulation is essential in pre-eclampsia. A falling platelet count is one of the earlier signs but the disease can rapidly progress to full DIC. At this stage, the pregnancy must be terminated and appropriate measures taken to correct the biochemical and haematological problems (57.2).

e) F Raised FDPs are not diagnostic in isolation (57.4).

58a) F The epidural space is open laterally via the intervertebral foraminae into the paravertebral spaces (58.1).

b) F The spinal dura mater and the arachnoid are closely adherent, forming the dural tube. The outer lining of the epidural space is the periosteum of the vertebral canal (58.1, 58.2).

c) F The spinal periosteum and the dura mater fuse at the foramen magnum, creating the intracranial dura mater (58.1, 58.2).

d) F The question concerns the epidural space rather than the dural sac. The dura ends at the second sacral segment in the adult but the space continues down to the sacro-coccygeal membrane (58.1).

e) F The epidural venous system communicates with the azygos system but has no valves (58.1, 58.2).

59 Pneumothorax is occasionally iatrogenic but may also be precipitated by a variety of diseases

Pneumothorax may be associated with:
a) Marfan's syndrome
b) asthma
c) interscalene brachial plexus block
d) fetal prematurity
e) emphysema

60 Dupuytren's contracture is often met clinically. Revising the associations of medical conditions is made easier by referring to 'list'-type texts.

Dupuytren's contracture is associated with:
a) cirrhosis of the liver
b) rheumatoid arthritis
c) sclerosing cholangitis
d) Hashimoto's disease
e) diabetes mellitus

References

59.1	Stoelting	p 640
59.2	Souhami & Moxham	p 490
59.3	Wildsmith	p 144
59.4	Kaplan	p 470
59.5	Synopsis	p 622
59.6	Practical Paed Problems	p 285
59.7	Davidson	p 397
60.1	Souhami & Moxham	p 644
60.2	Giles	p 625
60.3	OTM	p 9.88

59a) T Marfan's syndrome is a connective tissue defect inherited as an autosomal dominant. It is characterized by the patient being tall and thin with long, thin fingers. Clinical features include pectus excavatum, kyphoscoliosis and hyperextensible joints. Patients have a narrow, high arched palate and have a tendency to develop dissecting aneurysms of the ascending aorta, emphysema, lens dislocations, detached retina and pneumothorax. (59.1).

  b) T Pneumothorax is one of the less common conditions brought on by asthma (59.2).

  c) F The interscalene approach to the brachial plexus (Winnie's approach) is well above the dome of the pleura, unlike the supraclavicular or subclavian approaches (59.3, 59.4, 59.5).

  d) T Premature babies tend to develop the infant respiratory distress syndrome because of their inadequate production of surfactant. This gives a 'ground glass' appearance on chest X-ray and also leads to a high incidence of pneumothorax from IPPV. Over-vigorous resuscitation at birth can also cause pneumothorax. (59.6).

  e) T Patients with emphysema develop bullae on the lung surface. These air-filled cysts are really grossly overdistended terminal bronchioles. Occasionally the bullae rupture into the pleural space. They can also become so big that they themselves cause compression of the mediastinal structures – a kind of pseudo-pneumothorax (59.7).

60a) T A well known association (60.1).

  b) F There is no known association.

  c) T There is a very rare condition called multifocal fibrosclerosis which is characterized by the presence of two out of the following conditions: idiopathic mediastinal fibrosis, Riedel's thyroid fibrosis, Dupuytren's contracture and sclerosing cholangitis (60.2).

  d) F No connection exists.

  e) T Diabetes is one of the more common associations of Dupuytren's contracture and the incidence increases with the duration of the diabetes (60.3).

61 The causes of hypercapnia are legion, varying from the obvious to the obscure.

An elevated arterial partial pressure of carbon dioxide (Pa_{CO_2}) would be expected in:
a) pulmonary embolism
b) severe chronic bronchitis
c) the oliguric phase of renal failure
d) vomiting due to pyloric stenosis in an adult
e) diabetic ketoacidosis

62 Bronchial carcinoma is the most common malignancy in males and is responsible for 35 000 deaths every year.

Carcinoma of the bronchus may be associated with:
a) Cushing's syndrome
b) hyponatraemia
c) peripheral neuropathy
d) increased sensitivity to nondepolarizing muscle relaxants
e) hypercalcaemia

References
61.1   Nunn   p 384–385
61.2   Nunn   p 449
61.3   Zilva & Pannall   p 76–103

62.1   Muir   p 16.65–72
62.2   Kaplan   p 89
62.3   Katz & Kadis   p 622–626
62.4   Katz & Kadis   p 248

61a) F Pulmonary thromboembolism causes an increase in alveolar dead space which leads to a change in the alveolar-arterial CO_2 gradient. This might be thought to increase the Pa_{CO2} but in fact the remaining alveoli can easily cope with the CO_2 load, and the hyperventilation which usually accompanies pulmonary embolism means that subsequently the Pa_{CO2} is usually low (61.2).

b) T Elevated Pa_{CO2} is one of the signs of advancing respiratory failure in chronic obstructive pulmonary disease. 'Blue bloaters' are those patients whose normal drive to ventilation has been replaced by a ventilatory response to hypoxia (61.1).

c) F In the oliguric phase of acute renal failure the kidneys fail to excrete hydrogen ion. The hydrogen ion combines with bicarbonate to form carbonic acid and then carbon dioxide and water. The resulting metabolic acidosis is partly compensated by carbon dioxide being driven off by hyperventilation. The Pa_{CO2} does not rise and may fall in an attempt to return the pH to normal (61.4).

d) T Vomiting causes loss of both hydrogen ion from the stomach and bicarbonate from the duodenum. In pyloric stenosis, both adult and infant, the hydrogen ion is lost without the accompaniment of bicarbonate. A metabolic alkalosis follows and the compensatory mechanism is CO_2 retention, a respiratory acidosis, in an attempt to lower the pH (61.5).

e) F Diabetic ketoacidosis illustrates another condition in which there is a metabolic acidosis with a partly compensating respiratory alkalosis (61.3).

62 Carcinoma of the bronchus causes significant systemic disturbances in addition to local obstruction and invasion.

a) T Some tumours of the bronchus, especially oat-cell types, secrete ACTH. The result is Cushing's syndrome. (Harvey Cushing was a neurosurgeon in the 1920s) (62.1).

b) T Described in 1938 (62.2).

c) T This is not the myasthenic syndrome (see below) but a separate entity altogether which is identifiable by nerve conduction techniques (62.2).

d) T One of the best known associations of carcinoma of the bronchus is the Eaton–Lambert syndrome, alias the myasthenic syndrome. These unfortunates are exquisitely sensitive to the action of both depolarizing and nondepolarizing relaxants in terms of both the effective dose and the duration of action (62.3).

e) T Ectopic parathormone production can be responsible for hypercalcaemia (62.4).

63 The College guidelines for the Part 3 FRCAnaes state that candidates will not fail because of a poor knowledge of the history of anaesthesia (but they may have a hard time).

In a historical context:
a) Crawford Long used ether for anaesthesia in 1842
b) In 1847 James Simpson was the first to use chloroform in obstetrics.
c) Horace Wells extracted a tooth from Quincy Colton under nitrous oxide in 1844
d) Hannah Greener was the first recorded death from local anaesthesia
e) August Bier described spinal anaesthesia as a technique

64 Disorders of thyroid function are relatively common in patients presenting for surgery. Hypothyroidism is a notoriously difficult clinical diagnosis.

The following features suggest reduced thyroid function:
a) sensitivity to cold
b) tremor at rest
c) lower limb oedema
d) dry skin
e) macrocytic anaemia

References		
63.1	Sykes, vol 1	p 125–126
63.2	Moir	p 2–4
63.3	Sykes, vol 1	p 119–120
63.4	Sykes, vol 1	p 4
63.5	Moir	p 6
63.6	Sykes, vol 2	p 93
63.7	Synopsis	p 16
64.1	Davidson	p 630
64.2	Souhami & Moxham	p 695

63a) T Crawford Long gave the first ether anaesthetics in 1842. He failed to tell anyone for several years, but the claim is legitimate (63.1).

b) T Simpson gave the first obstetric anaesthetic using ether in January 1847, and using chloroform in November the same year (63.2).

c) F It was nitrous oxide in 1844, it was Colton and Wells, but the anaesthetist was Colton and the pationt was Wells (63.3).

d) F Hannah Greener was a 15 year old girl who was the subject of the first recorded general anaesthetic death, from chloroform in 1848. This was long before local anaesthesia was introduced in 1884 (63.4, 63.6).

e) T August Bier is remembered for the intravenous regional anaesthetic technique which bears his name but he also gave the first deliberate spinal anaesthetics in 1899. Note that Corning had given accidental spinals in 1885 but this method proved unreliable (63.5, 63.7).

64 Hypothyroidism is an insidious condition which may come on over decades. The symptoms are so nonspecific that the prevalence is unknown.

a) T Sensitivity to cold is one of the most frequent symptoms at presentation (64.1).

b) F Tremor may be a sign of hyperthyroid states (64.1).

c) F The 'oedema' of myxoedema is not really oedema but a deposition of a mucopolysaccharide in the subcutaneous tissues which does not pit on pressure. Although this substance is often pre-tibial, the face is a more common site of deposition (64.1).

d) T Dry skin is one of the classical features of the disease (64.1).

e) F The anaemia of hypothyroidism is usually normocytic, normochromic as a result of marrow hypocellularity, but may occasionally be macrocytic because of the association of myxoedema with pernicious anaemia (64.2).

65 Obstructive jaundice and the anaesthetic problems associated with it are as common in the examinations as they are in the operating theatre.

Obstructive jaundice secondary to gallstones is associated with:
a) excess urine urobilinogen
b) generalized pruritus
c) a painless palpable gall bladder
d) a high plasma concentration of unconjugated bilirubin
e) a high plasma alkaline phosphatase

66 The vast majority of anaesthetics include nitrous oxide without any thought for the consequences associated with this gas which is far from being innocuous.

Nitrous oxide:
a) is below its critical temperature at room temperature
b) will support combustion
c) interferes with the metabolism of folic acid
d) does not increase intracranial pressure in the presence of space occupying lesions
e) was discovered by Humphrey Davy

References

65.1	Sherlock	p 235–239
66.1	Recent Advances 16	p 20
66.2	Recent Advances 16	p 33
66.3	Synopsis	p 511
66.4	Synopsis	p 4

65a) F If obstruction is total there will be no urobilinogen at all in the urine because none can be secreted into the bowel for reabsorption and later renal excretion. Even if obstruction is subtotal there will certainly not be an excess over normal (65.1).

b) T Pruritus is one of the differentiating signs between hepatic and post-hepatic causes of jaundice. Pruritus only occurs if bilirubin has been conjugated before systemic absorption (65.1).

c) F Painless enlargement of the gall bladder tends to be associated with the gradual onset of obstruction because of malignant disease rather than gall stones (65.1).

d) F While the plasma levels of bilirubin do rise in obstructive jaundice, it is the conjugated form which predominates, because hepatic function is maintained until quite late in the disease (65.1).

e) T Alkaline phosphatase concentrations of three times normal are not uncommon (65.1).

66 Nitrous oxide was once thought to be a totally benign vehicle which took no part in metabolism. This is not so.

a) T The critical temperature for a gas is the temperature above which it cannot be liquefied by pressure alone. The critical pressure is the pressure required to cause liquefaction at the critical temperature. The critical temperature for nitrous oxide is 36.43 $^{\circ}$C. Thus it remains liquid when stored under pressure in cylinders at room temperature (66.1).

b) T Nitrous oxide will support combustion, decomposing into nitrogen and oxygen at 450°C (66.1).

c) T There have been a number of detailed reviews of this action in the anaesthetic press recently (66.2).

d) F All other things being equal, nitrous oxide does not increase the intracranial pressure in the normal brain, but it may do so in the presence of a space-occupying lesion or oedema (66.3).

e) F Humphrey Davy is renowned for his observation that the pain of a dental abscess was reduced when breathing the gas and for his suggestion that it might have a use in surgery, but he took the matter no further. Joseph Priestley discovered the gas in 1772, not Davy (66.4).

67 Asthma is defined by The American Thoracic Society as 'a disease characterized by increased responsiveness of the bronchi to various stimuli, manifested by widespread narrowing of the airways that changes in severity either spontaneously or as the result of treatment'.

Asthma:
a) is associated with Churg–Strauss syndrome
b) may be treated with sympathomimetic agents effectively
c) has a peak age of onset of 10 years
d) may be triggered by respiratory infection
e) is responsible for about 5000 deaths per year in the United Kingdom

68 A patient in chronic hepatocellular failure may have:
a) a high plasma urea
b) gynaecomastia
c) hyponatraemia
d) a lower dose requirement for nondepolarizing muscle relaxants
e) a clotting defect which responds to oral phytomenadione

References

67.1   Souhami & Moxham   p 485–492

68.1   Sherlock   p 87
68.2   Sherlock   p 91
68.3   Sherlock   p 122
68.4   Miller   p 398–399
68.5   Sherlock   p 53
68.6   Nimmo & Smith   p 906–907

67a) T Churg–Strauss syndrome is one of a group of eosinophilic syndromes which are associated with asthma (67.1).
  b) T Sympathomimetic amines are the mainstay of treatment (67.1).
  c) F The peak age of onset of asthma is less than five years (67.4).
  d) T Other triggers include exercise, cold air, fumes and laughter (67.1).
  e) F This figure is too high. The mortality rate per annum is around 2000 (67.1).

68 The causes of hepatocellular failure are many, from alcohol, drug effects, infection, to tumour. The end result is the same, that is to say, a patient in biochemical turmoil.
  a) F Urea is a product of hepatic metabolism but, despite this, the liver capacity for urea manufacture is enormous and so the plasma urea is usually normal until the terminal stages of liver failure, at which point it may become low (68.1).
  b) T Gynaecomastia is one of the cardinal signs of chronic liver disease. It results from the failure of the liver to eliminate the sex hormones. The water excess of hepatic failure is often treated with spironolactone, which can itself cause gynaecomastia (68.2).
  c) T Hyponatraemia is dilutional (68.3).
  d) F Patients with hepatocellular failure are usually water overloaded. They may also have abnormal plasma protein concentrations. The combination of these two means that the volume of distribution of the relaxants is increased compared to normal, and therefore the dose necessary to produce relaxation may be increased. Excretion will be prolonged (68.4, 68.6).
  e) F Note that the stem says 'oral'. Vitamin K_1 is absorbed from the gut in association with the bile acids. In hepatocellular failure, bile acids are not excreted into the gut and there will be poor vitamin K absorption. The usual route for administration is intramuscular, since it is a more reliable way of improving the coagulation state (68.5).

69 The design and function of anaesthetic equipment forms part of the scope of the Part 3 FRCAnaes examination.

The Flu otec Mark IV vaporizer:
a) is a temperature compensated, variable bypass vaporizer
b) delivers relatively constant vapour concentrations despite variations in gas flow
c) could be used for isoflurane without recalibration
d) is designed to function even when tipped away from vertical
e) has two bypass channels

70 Clinical biochemistry questions require the application of logic before the answers are attempted. Take your time.

A serum bicarbonate concentration of 11 mmol/l would be found in:
a) metabolic acidosis
b) respiratory acidosis with metabolic compensation
c) respiratory alkalosis with metabolic compensation
d) metabolic alkalosis with respiratory compensation
e) metabolic acidosis with respiratory compensation

References		
69.1	Ward	p 77–82
69.2	Synopsis	p 172
70.1	Davenport	p 71
70.2	Davenport	p 77–79
70.3	Davenport	p 89–91

69a) T The temperature compensation device, a bimetallic strip, is on the inlet side of the bypass chamber. The control valve alters the splitting ratio between the bypass and the vaporization chamber (69.1).

b) T The Mark IV Flu otec on a setting of 5% gives 3.5% at 14 l/min gas flow and 5.5% at one l/min. The Mark III version was closer to linear (69.1).

c) T The SVP, boiling point and molecular weights of halothane and isoflurane are so similar that it would indeed be possible to use a halothane vaporizer for isoflurane without recalibration, provided that the vaporizer had either not been used before or been well washed out, to remove the thymol. Not a sensible idea, however (69.2).

d) T The design allows the vaporizer to be tipped without liquid halothane coming out of the bypass channel, unlike the Mark III (69.1).

e) T In the 'off' position there are two bypass channels open. When the vaporizer is turned 'on', even at a zero setting, one of these is closed off and gas is diverted to the temperature compensated bypass (69.1).

70a) T The characteristics of uncompensated metabolic acidosis are: normal Pa_{CO_2}, low pH and low bicarbonate (70.1).

b) F Respiratory acidosis follows from a rise in the Pa_{CO_2}. This increases the bicarbonate concentration because of the increased carbonic acid concentration. The rise in Pa_{CO_2} elevates the renal reabsorption of bicarbonate, restoring the pH toward normal but increasing the concentration of bicarbonate even further (70.3).

c) T Respiratory alkalosis follows a fall in the Pa_{CO_2} from hyperventilation. Bicarbonate is converted to carbon dioxide to compensate and the pH rises. The fall in Pa_{CO_2} reduces the renal tubular reabsorption of bicarbonate and the bicarbonate concentration falls even further (70.3).

d) F In metabolic alkalosis the pH rises. The increased pH depresses respiration and the Pa_{CO_2} is elevated. The increase in Pa_{CO_2} raises the pH but also increases the bicarbonate concentration (70.2).

e) T The decreased pH of metabolic acidosis stimulates respiration which drives off CO_2 and restores the pH again. The fall in Pa_{CO_2} causes a fall in bicarbonate concentration, which is already low in metabolic acidosis (70.2).

71 Journal articles aim to present new ideas in a scientific way. A knowledge of basic statistical methods is essential if articles are not to be taken at face value but criticized constructively.

The standard deviation:
a) cannot be calculated for discontinuous data
b) indicates the first point of inflection on a normal distribution curve
c) defines the limits of normality
d) is the square root of the variance
e) indicates the spread of results about the mean

72 The following are signs of lower small bowel obstruction:
a) nausea and vomiting
b) abdominal distension
c) rumbling low grade bowel sounds
d) dullness in the flanks
e) constant abdominal pain

References

71.1   Swinscow   p 7–15

72.1   Jones   p 131

71 Calculation of the standard deviation (SD) for a set of data is one of the simplest statistical manoeuvres and has a multitude of applications.
  a) F Discontinuous data is data that is confined to whole numbers or discrete blocks. The standard deviation calculated from this is just as valid as for continuous data (71.1).
  b) T One SD either side of the mean will indicate the point where the rate of change of gradient of the curve changes from negative to positive.
  c) F What is normal? It is only a statistical convention that any result falling outside 3 SDs can be treated as outside the population under consideration (71.1).
  d) T One way of calculating standard deviation (71.1).
  e) T A definition of standard deviation (71.1).

72a) T Nausea and vomiting occur with almost every intra-abdominal event (72.1).
  b) T The lower down the gut the obstruction occurs, the greater will be the distension (72.1).
  c) F The bowel sounds of intestinal obstruction are high pitched and 'tinkling' in nature (72.1).
  d) F Dullness in the flanks is a sign more of free fluid than of an intraluminal problem (72.1).
  e) F The pain of intestinal obstruction, as with any other obstructed hollow organ, is 'colicky' i.e. it comes in waves. It is not constant in nature (72.1).

73 Read the question carefully. Do not jump at the weight loss element without realising that the qualification of appetite makes the question very specific.

Loss of weight with normal or increased appetite may be found in:
a) carcinoma of stomach
b) thyrotoxicosis
c) diabetes mellitus
d) Addison's disease
e) pulmonary tuberculosis

74 Examination of the arterial system is one of the first things taught in medical school. While the finer detail may be the province of a cardiologist, medicine to the standard of medical school exit qualification is expected for the FRCAnaes diploma.

A small pulse pressure may be found in:
a) aortic stenosis
b) mitral stenosis
c) patent ductus arteriosus
d) beri-beri
e) cor pulmonale

References

73.1	OTM	p 12.148
73.2	OTM	p 10.41
73.3	OTM	p 9.53
73.4	OTM	p 5.288
73.5	Souhami & Moxham	p 706
74.1	Braunwald	p 924
74.2	Braunwald	p 993
74.3	Braunwald	p 1027
74.4	Braunwald	p 1055
74.5	Braunwald	p 1606
74.6	Braunwald	p 786–787

73a) F Carcinoma of the stomach usually presents late. There may be little by the way of symptoms until the onset of anorexia and weight loss, by which time any operation will be palliative (73.1).
  b) T Thyrotoxicosis causes loss of weight with sustained appetite (73.2).
  c) T Diabetes is classically a wasting disease but the appetite is variable. The patient may be anorexic but often has cravings for sugary drinks and food (73.3).
  d) F Addison's disease, adrenal failure, usually includes weight loss in the presentation (73.4).
  e) F Patients with pulmonary tuberculosis of long standing lose weight and have a reduced appetite (73.5).

74 Note that the stem says 'may be' rather than 'is'. Some texts use 'narrow' where others use 'small' when referring to pulse pressure.
  a) T The pulse pressure in aortic stenosis is low, with the arterial pressure wave being small and sustained (74.1).
  b) T The pulse pressure in mitral stenosis depends upon the left ventricular function. If this is normal then the pulse pressure will be normal. If the ventricular function is reduced, the stroke volume is reduced and the pulse pressure will be reduced. Again, the operative words are 'may be' (74.2).
  c) F A patent ductus arteriosus is an open channel between the pulmonary and systemic circulations. Usually the pressure in the pulmonary vasculature is lower than that in the aorta. Therefore the duct provides a run-off channel and the pulse pressure is low (74.1, 74.2, 74.3).
  d) F Beri-beri, the chronic deficiency of thiamine, causes high-output cardiac failure, high venous return and low systemic vascular resistance. The pulse pressure is increased as it would be in most hyperdynamic states (74.4).
  e) F Cor pulmonale is the name given to right ventricular failure as a consequence of pulmonary hypertension. There is some debate about the involvement of the left ventricle. There are rare cases of left ventricular failure in cor pulmonale but the aetiology is uncertain. More commonly, left ventricular function is normal, as is the pulse pressure. Retention of carbon dioxide tends to cause a fall in systemic vascular resistance (74.5, 74.6).

ꞈctopic hormone production is a feature of many tumours both endocrine and non-endocrino.

The following substances may be secreted inappropriately by tumours:
a) a parathyroid hormone-like substance
b) 5-hydroxytryptamine
c) 5-hydroxytryptophane
d) somatostatin
e) vasoactive intestinal peptide

76 The porphyrias are an intriguing group of inborn errors of metabolism. Rare though they may be, except in South Africa, some of their associations and interactions are of great practical relevance.

Barbiturate anaesthesia is considered safe in:
a) porphyria cutanea tarda
b) acute intermittent porphyria
c) variegate porphyria
d) hereditary cuproporphyria
e) erythropoietic protoporphyria

References		
75.1	Muir	p 16.70–77
75.2	Giles	p 601
75.3	Giles	p 1110–1112
76.1	Stoelting	p 529–531
76.2	BJA (1992) 68	p 230

75 Tumours may secrete a variety of substances, the commonest of which are ACTH, ADH and steroids.
   a) T Parathyroid tumours would be expected to secrete parathyroid hormone, and do. Parathyroid hormone-like substances can also be secreted by oat-cell tumours of the lung (75.2, 75.3).
   b) T 5-HT is secreted by carcinoid tumours, especially if there are extensive liver metastases. This is the factor responsible for the flushing and paroxysmal blood pressure changes of the carcinoid syndrome (75.1).
   c) T 5-hydroxytryptophane is the precursor of 5-HT (see above). Bronchial carcinoids may secrete this rather than 5-HT itself because they lack carboxylase in endodermal tissue to convert 5-hydroxytryptophane into 5-HT (75.1).
   d) T Pancreatic tumours can (rarely) secrete somatostatin (75.2).
   e) T Non-beta cell tumours of the pancreas may secrete VIP (vasoactive intestinal peptide), giving rise to a syndrome of watery diarrhoea and achlorhydria (75.2).

76 The porphyrias are abnormalities of haem synthesis. The complex interplay of the various enzyme defects and oversecretions is too extensive to detail here. Basically, as far as anaesthesia is concerned, the hepatic porphyrias can be a problem whereas the cutaneous ones are less so.
   a) T Porphyria cutanea tarda is the only form of hepatic porphyria not associated with neurological deficit. It is caused by reduced activity of uroporphyrinogen decarboxylase. The patients have photosensitivity, a friable skin and may give a history of alcohol abuse. Anaesthesia is said not to be a problem, though there is often associated chronic liver disease due to accumulation of porphyrins causing hepatocellular necrosis (76.1).
   b) F Acute intermittent porphyria is the classic condition, with 'port wine' urine on exposure to light. The defects appear to be both a decrease in uroporphyrinogen synthetase activity and an increase in the activity of aminolaevulinic acid synthetase. These give rise to excess porphobilinogen. The patients present with intermittent abdominal pain, demyelinating neurological deficits and peculiar behaviour. There are a number of drugs which are said to precipitate an attack; the barbiturates form one large group, the benzodiazepines another. In general the opioids are safe. Etomidate is not. So far there is little information about the use of propofol (76.1, 76.2).
   c) F The clinical features include photosensitivity, skin friability and neurological deficits. The barbiturates should be avoided (76.1).
   d) F The management of hereditary ouproporphyria is similar to that for acute intermittent porphyria (76.1).
   e) T Erythropoietic protoporphyrias show some of the features of erythropoietic uroporphyria but with survival into adulthood. There are no adverse effects from barbiturates (76.1).

77 The following factors predispose to postoperative renal failure:
   a) prolonged intraoperative hypotension
   b) administration of radiographic contrast media
   c) septic shock
   d) preoperative pneumonia
   e) obstructive jaundice

78 The unwanted and toxic effects of the cardiac glycosides will frequently
be met in all three parts of the anaesthetic diploma examination.

Overdosage with digitalis alkaloids:
   a) causes a prolonged P–R interval
   b) causes a prolonged Q–T interval
   c) causes diarrhoea
   d) causes neuralgia
   e) frusemide is part of the treatment

References

77.1 Miller   p 1170–1180

78.1 Rowlands 2   p 220–222
78.2 Goodman & Gilman   p 832–835

77a) T Prolonged hypotension causes acute tubular dysfunction and glomerular failure. This is a classic cause of acute renal failure (77.1).

b) T The mechanism of causation of renal failure by contrast media is unclear (77.1).

c) T The presence of septic shock predisposes to the development of postoperative renal failure, by reducing renal perfusion and increasing the delivery of toxins to the glomerulus and tubule (77.1).

d) F Excluding parlous states where severe hypoxia exists there will be no connection.

e) T Obstructive jaundice is another classic cause of postoperative renal failure (hepatorenal syndrome), although the mechanism is not clear (77.1).

78 Digitalis alkaloids (cardiac glycosides) inhibit the cellular sodium ionic pump, which explain some of their effects.

a) F Digoxin and the other digitalis alkaloids cause prolongation rather than shortening of the P–R interval, to the extent of either first degree heart block or even type I second degree heart block (Wenckebach type) (78.1).

b) T Short Q–T interval is a sign of effective therapy rather than toxicity (78.1).

c) T Diarrhoea may be the presenting feature of glycoside toxicity (78.2).

d) T The neuralgia of glycoside toxicity may mimic trigeminal neuralgia (78.2).

e) F The toxicity of cardiac glycosides is exacerbated by hypokalaemia and reduced by potassium administration. Any diuretic which causes potassium loss should be withdrawn along with the offending alkaloid (78.2).

79 Minimum alveolar concentration (MAC) has a specific definition which is a prerequisite to answering this question.

Minimum alveolar concentration (MAC):
a) varies with age
b) is more than 100% for nitrous oxide
c) is measured with 30% oxygen in nitrous oxide as the carrier gas mixture
d) indicates the concentration necessary for induction of anaesthesia
e) is an ED$_{95}$ for the drug in question

80 Some of the rarer complications of pregnancy give no warning of their onset. If 'HELLP' syndrome is unfamiliar, read the reference first.

'HELLP' syndrome in pregnancy may cause:
a) arterial hypotension
b) jaundice
c) haemolytic anaemia
d) hypoglycaemia
e) polyuria

References

79.1	BJA (1990) 65	p 527–536
79.2	Nimmo & Smith	p 36
80.1	BJA (1991) 66	p 513–515

79 Minimal alveolar concentration is a measure of true anaesthetic vapour potency. It allows comparison of one vapour with another. MAC is defined as 'the minimum alveolar concentration which, in steady state, will prevent movement in response to abdominal skin incision in 50% of unpremedicated ASA 1 patients when used as sole agent in oxygen'.
   a) T It is no surprise that the amount of a drug necessary for any effect varies with the age and fitness of the patient (79.1).
   b) T The reason why awareness-free anaesthesia cannot be guaranteed without additional supplementation (79.2).
   c) F MAC must be measured in oxygen only (79.2).
   d) F MAC is defined at a steady state, not during the unstable conditions of induction. The solubility of an agent in blood will give a much better indication of its induction characteristics (79.2).
   e) F MAC is the ED_{50} of the agent not ED_{95} (79.2).

80 HELLP syndrome was described in 1982 as the most severe and dangerous form of pre-eclampsia. The acronym stands for Haemolytic anaemia, Elevated Liver enzymes and Low Platelets.
   a) F It is a variation of pre-eclampsia and so presents with hypertension rather than hypotension (80.1).
   b) T Jaundice results from disturbed liver function (80.1).
   c) T Part of the acronym for the name (80.1) as described above.
   d) T Patients with HELLP syndrome develop sudden and severe hypoglycaemia, especially under anaesthesia and later in the intensive care unit. Presumably this too is a reflection of deranged liver function (80.1).
   e) F Acute renal failure with oliguria is more likely as a result of hypovolaemia, deposition of red cell fragments, haemoglobinuria and disseminated intravascular coagulation (80.1).

81 Post dural puncture headache (PDPH) has been referred to extensively
    in the anaesthetic press as the types of needle point available for
    subarachnoid block have diversified.

    The incidence of post dural puncture headache is decreased:
    a) with decreasing age
    b) in pregnancy
    c) by the use of smaller needles
    d) by the use of conical-tipped needles
    e) if the patient lies supine for 24 hours after the procedure

82 **High cardiac output may be caused by:**
    a) hypovolaemic shock
    b) thyrotoxicosis
    c) a large arteriovenous malformation
    d) aortic aneurysm
    e) Paget's disease of bone

References		
81.1	BJA (1991) 66	p 596–607
82.1	Synopsis	p 745
82.2	Stoelting	p 478–482
82.3	Miller	p 1774
82.4	Stoelting	p 638

81a) F Younger patients have a very high incidence of PDPH, possibly because of their mobility, possibly because of the compliance of the cranial and lumbar spaces (81.1).

b) F There is debate as to whether the incidence is increased in pregnancy, but it is certainly not reduced (81.1).

c) T Unfortunately, smaller needles are also more difficult to use and therefore there is a higher failure rate and a higher rate of multiple tap (81.1).

d) T The Whitacre and more recent Sprötte needles tend to part the dural fibres rather than cutting them, at least that is the theory (81.1).

e) F 24-hour bed rest is custom and practice but seems to make no difference, thus the patient may as well mobilize as soon as the block wears off (81.1).

82a) F In hypovolaemic shock, circulating volume is reduced and venous return is lessened. This reduced preload causes a low cardiac output (82.1).

b) T Thyrotoxicosis is an extreme version of the hyperthyroid state. Hyperdynamic circulation, including a high cardiac output, is one of the most obvious signs (82.2).

c) T Large arteriovenous malformations provide a low-resistance pathway from the arterial to the venous circulations. This can be so large as to require a high cardiac output to maintain perfusion of the remainder of the body (82.3).

d) F There is no association.

e) T Paget's disease is a condition in which deposition and resorption of bone mineral are abnormally high. The increase in bone metabolism can be so high that the cardiac output rises to match it (82.4).

83 In prolapse of the L4/5 intervertebral disc causing sciatica:
a) there are diminished quadriceps tendon reflexes
b) urinary incontinence is an indication for urgent surgery
c) there is anaesthesia of the medial aspect of the calf
d) there may be scoliosis
e) the treatment of first choice is plaster of Paris jacket

84 MAC values may vary alarmingly from source to source. Answers within 0.2% are acceptable here. In the actual examination there may be no leeway in the MCQ. That which agrees with the computer marking system will gain the mark.

Anaesthetic vapours have the following values for minimum alveolar concentration (MAC):
a) halothane 0.7%
b) enflurane 1.6%
c) isoflurane 1.8%
d) desflurane 6%
e) sevoflurane 2%

References

83.1	Gray	p 1123
83.2	Wildsmith	p 156
83.3	Gray	p 1143
83.4	Gray	p 1420–1421
83.5	OTM	p 16.82
83.6	OTM	p 21.113
84.1	Dunnill & Colvin	p 5
84.2	BJA (1990) 65	p 527–536

83 Think long and hard about each completion. The L4 root will probably not be compressed by an L4/5 protrusion (83.1, 83.2). The symptoms of 'sciatica' tend to be from S1 or L5 compression.

a) **F** The quadriceps are innervated by the femoral nerve, L2,3,4. There is no involvement of these nerve roots (83.3, 83.4, 83.5).

b) **T** Urinary incontinence is a sign of cauda equina compression, indicating a large central prolapse of such severity that the blood supply to the roots is compromized. Urgent surgery may save the day (83.6).

c) **F** The medial aspect of the calf is innervated by the saphenous nerve, a branch of the femoral which is not involved in this case. (83.2, 83.3, 83.5).

d) **T** Scoliosis may be the cause of the condition or it may be the result of muscle spasm induced by pain (83.5).

e) **F** The first line treatment is rest and analgesia (83.5).

84a) T This is essential knowledge (84.1).

b) **T** As above (84.1).

c) **F** The correct value is 1.2% (84.1).

d) **T** The two agents in this and the next completion are under investigation at the moment. They promise to go some way towards the so called 'ideal' anaesthetic agent (84.2).

e) **T** Note that these MAC values are approximate at present (84.2).

Salicylate preparations are widely consumed with and without medical advice. Acetyl salicylic acid has an intriguing variety of actions.

Aspirin in low dosage (up to 150 mg per day):
a) inhibits platelet thromboxane synthetase
b) inactivates platelet cyclo-oxygenase
c) blocks production of thromboxane A_2
d) inactivates cyclo-oxygenase in vascular endothelium
e) causes mild vasodilatation

86 **The following drugs are extensively metabolized in the liver:**
a) nifedipine
b) enalapril
c) ketamine
d) diltiazem
e) etomidate

References

85.1	Goodman & Gilman	p 1325
85.2	BJA (1991) 66	p 1–4
86.1	Dundee, Clarke & McCaughey	p 413–414
86.2	Dundee, Clarke & McCaughey	p 430
86.3	Recent Advances 15	p 35–37

85 Until the 1970's, aspirin was thought to be merely an anti- inflammatory, antipyretic analgesic. It now has other applications, such as reduction of platelet stickiness.
   a) F Aspirin blocks production of thromboxane A_2 but not by inhibition of thromboxane synthetase (85.1).
   b) T Cyclo-oxygenase is inactivated by acetylation of the active site on the enzyme. This is permanent, hence the duration of the effect in any individual platelet (85.1).
   c) T Cyclo-oxygenase produces the cyclic endoperoxide precursor of thromboxane A_2 (TxA_2). If cyclo-oxygenase is blocked then TxA_2 will not be made (85.1).
   d) F The cyclo-oxygenase of the vascular endothelium is blocked by aspirin but not in low doses. The dose required for this effect is in the order of 1–1.5 g per 24 hours (85.2).
   e) T TxA_2 is a vasoconstrictor, the inhibition of which by aspirin will cause mild vasodilatation (85.2).

86 Drug metabolism by the liver may take several forms. There may be conversion from an inactive to an active form, or from the active to the inactive form, or from water insoluble to water soluble forms before excretion.
   a) F First pass liver extraction of nifedipine is small and some 85% is excreted in the urine (86.1).
   b) T Enalapril is a prodrug. The active drug is enalaprilat. Both are excreted unchanged in the urine but the conversion from one to the other is liver dependent (86.2).
   c) T Ketamine is metabolized in the liver to a wide variety of products (86.3).
   d) T While diltiazem is excreted unchanged, the hepatic first pass effect is extensive (86.1).
   e) T There is extensive hepatic hydrolysis of etomidate and less than 2% is excreted unchanged (86.3).

87 The catecholamine output which results from laryngoscopy and intubation has been the subject of many research projects. The mechanism is slowly becoming more clearly understood.

The pressor response to laryngoscopy and intubation can be attenuated by:
a) intravenous fentanyl 1 µg/kg
b) captopril
c) lignocaine surface spray to the larynx and trachea
d) nasal nitroglycerin
e) diltiazem

88 **With respect to the cranial nerves:**
a) the maxillary nerve passes through the foramen ovale in the base of the skull
b) the jugular foramen transmits the XIth (spinal accessory) nerve
c) the Vth (trigeminal) nerve has no motor component
d) the masseter muscles are supplied from the VIIth (facial) nerve
e) the VIIth (facial) nerve has no branches before its exit from the stylo-mastoid foramen

References

87.1	Synopsis	p 218
87.2	Anaesthesia (1990) 45	p 243
87.3	Anaesthesia (1990) 45	p 289
88.1	Gray	p 1103–1106
88.2	Gray	p 359
88.3	Gray	p 1099–1100
88.4	Gray	p 1107–1109

87 The pressor response to laryngoscopy and intubation may add to cardiovascular morbidity. Unmodified, the arterial pressure and heart rate increase dramatically.

a) F Fentanyl only attenuates the pressor response in doses greater than 5 µg/kg (87.3).

b) T Captopril is an inhibitor of angiotensin converting enzyme. Unfortunately, in the study cited the arterial pressure fell dramatically (87.2).

c) T Adequate local anaesthesia of the larynx will attenuate the response (87.1).

d) T The response is muted (87.1).

e) T The response is muted (87.3).

88a) F The mandibular branch of the trigeminal nerve comes through the foramen ovale, the maxillary branch comes through the foramen rotundum, just anterior and medial to the foramen ovale (88.1).

b) T There are also other contents of note (88.2).

c) F The trigeminal is the major sensory nerve of the face but has a motor component which joins the mandibular branch beyond the Gasserian ganglion (see d) (88.3).

d) F The masseters are supplied by the motor component of the trigeminal (88.3).

e) F The facial nerve runs a complex course from the brain, through the internal auditory meatus, an acute bend in the petrous temporal bone, and gives off several branches before it leaves the stylo-mastoid foramen. These are the external, greater superficial and lesser superficial petrosal nerves (88.4).

89 Newts and tadpoles are time honoured examples of species in which pressure reversal of anaesthesia may be demonstrated. The basis for this effect is less well remembered.

Pressure reversal of anaesthetic action:
a) cannot be demonstrated in mammals
b) can be explained by the multi-site expansion hypothesis
c) explains the relationship between MAC and the oil/gas partition coefficient
d) can only be observed with inhalational agents
e) only occurs in excess of 200 atmospheres

90 With regard to pharmacokinetics:
a) plasma clearance is independent of the concentration of drug
b) the volume of distribution may be greater than the total body water
c) protein binding in the plasma may reduce the volume of distribution
d) the plasma half-life gives an indication of the duration of action
e) in the doses usually employed, thiopentone has zero order kinetics

---

References

89.1 Dundee, Clarke & McCaughey   p 85–89

90.1 Recent Advances 15   p 27–33

89 Despite prolonged investigation of the action of general anaesthetic agents, there is still no unified theory to explain our daily anaesthetic practice.
   a) F Pressure reversal is demonstrable in mammals, including man (89.1).
   b) T The multi-site expansion hypothesis suggests that there are a number of sites on the cell membrane which change shape under the influence of different drugs, with differing effects. These changes can be reversed with pressure. This is an expanded and updated version of the critical volume hypothesis (89.1).
   c) F There is a linear relationship between the MAC of an agent and its oil/gas partition coefficient. This is not explained by, nor does it explain, pressure reversal (89.1).
   d) F Pressure reversal is also observable when non-inhalational agents are used (89.1).
   e) F Pressure reversal occurs at low pressure, but is difficult to observe until higher pressures are reached (89.1).

90a) T The plasma clearance is a measure of the volume of plasma cleared of drug in unit time. It is measured in ml/min or ml/h. The concentration of the drug is irrelevant (90.1).
   b) T The volume of distribution is derived from the plasma concentration of the drug. High fat solubility may increase this volume above the volume of total body water by extraction from the plasma (90.1).
   c) T If there is significant protein binding then drug is kept in the plasma rather than being distributed to other compartments, reducing the volume of distribution (90.1).
   d) F The plasma half-life only measures the fall in concentration of the drug with time. The effects of the drug are unrelated to this because of factors such as receptor binding and fat depot deposition (90.1).
   e) F Zero order kinetics imply that an enzyme system has been saturated with drug and this limits the rate of excretion. This only occurs with thiopentone at high dose and over a prolonged period (90.1).

91 Peripheral vascular resistance is affected by physiological factors and extraneously administered agents.

Peripheral vascular resistance is increased by:
a) generalized sympathetic activity
b) the injection of renin
c) kallikrein activation
d) sodium citrate
e) injection of adrenaline

92 Patients suffering from diabetes mellitus frequently present for surgery. The pathology of the disease leads to abnormal responses to anaesthesia and surgery.

In insulin dependent diabetes mellitus:
a) the insulin requirement increases in the first trimester of pregnancy
b) gastric emptying may be prolonged
c) there may be painless myocardial ischaemia
d) insulin requirement is increased by anaesthesia
e) insulin requirement is increased by surgery

References		
91.1	Guyton	p 194–202
91.2	Guyton	p 211–214
91.3	Guyton	p 191–192
92.1	Stoelting	p 787
92.2	Stoelting	p 522–525

91a) T Generalized sympathetic activity implies nervous as well as hormonal influence. Peripheral vascular resistance increases, mainly due to the action of noradrenaline (91.1, 91.2).

b) T Renin, acting as the initiator of the renin-angiotensin control mechanism, causes peripheral constriction (albeit indirectly) (91.2).

c) F Kallikrein is activated by similar insults to those which precipitate platelet aggregation. Activated kallikrein acts upon alpha-1 globulins to produce kallidin, which is converted to bradykinin. Bradykinin is a potent vasodilator (91.3).

d) F Citrate is a vasodilator, a fact which may assume importance during massive blood transfusion (91.3).

e) F Adrenaline possesses both alpha and beta actions. It has a vasoconstrictor influence on skin and gut but vasodilates skeletal muscle, an effect which predominates, thus causing a fall in PVR. (91.1, 91.2).

92a) F Insulin requirement falls in the first trimester of pregnancy before rising again in the second. There is a major fall in requirement in the puerperium (92.1).

b) T Diabetic patients tend to develop an autonomic neuropathy of which one effect can be delayed gastric emptying (92.2).

c) T The autonomic neuropathy (see above) may also include the cardiac nerve supply, eliminating or reducing cardiac pain (92.2).

d) F Although the effects of anaesthesia and surgery are difficult to separate, anaesthesia itself ooomo to have no consistent hyperglycaemic effect (92.2).

e) T Surgery tends to cause a rise in blood glucose, increasing the insulin needs of the patient throughout the perioperative period (92.2).

93 Cardiac output may be measured by invasive or non-invasive methods. Non-invasive methods are improving rapidly but remain less accurate than invasive methods, most of which involve the use of pulmonary artery flotation catheters.

When measuring the cardiac output:
a) thermodilution is an example of an indirect Fick method
b) ballistocardiography is a non-invasive method
c) analysis of the radial pulse may be used in the characteristic impedance method
d) blood flow in the bronchial and thebesian veins causes inaccuracy in indicator dilution methods
e) the direct Fick method can only be used with oxygen as the indicator

94 The Mapleson classification of anaesthesia breathing systems should be held in every reputable departmental library.

In the Mapleson classification of anaesthetic systems:
a) when breathing spontaneously with a 'D' system, the fresh gas flow must be three times minute volume to avoid a rise in Pa_{CO2}
b) when breathing spontaneously with the 'A' system, the fresh gas flow may be less than minute volume without causing a rise in Pa_{CO2}
c) when used for spontaneous breathing, the 'B' system requires a fresh gas flow of 2.5 times minute volume to avoid a rise in Pa_{CO2}
d) during spontaneous breathing with the 'D' system, the fresh gas flow must be greater than the peak inspiratory flow rate
e) during controlled ventilation with the 'D' system, the Pa_{CO2} depends upon the fresh gas flow alone

References

93.1 Scurr, Feldman & Soni   p 82–103

94.1 BJA (1954) 26   p 223ff.
94.2 Nimmo & Smith   p 328

93 There are a variety of more or less accurate and more or less cumbersome methods of cardiac output measurement. Few have made the transition from laboratory to bedside. The direct Fick methods depend upon the passage (unchanged) through the heart of a measurable substance or a physical property.

  a) F The thermodilution method is a direct Fick method, the passage of a bolus of cold fluid from the right atrium to the pulmonary artery (93.1).

  b) T Ballistocardiography measures the movement of the whole body caused by each cardiac contraction. It has been used to measure the cardiac output in a whale (93.1).

  c) T The characteristic impedance method measures the velocity of a peripheral pulse and analyses its waveform. It is not accurate and cannot be used at the bedside (93.1).

  d) T The bronchial and thebesian vessels recirculate indicator from the left to the right side of the heart rather than through the peripheral circulation. This leads to inaccuracies in measurement of dye concentration (93.1).

  e) F Laboratory 'direct' Fick methods use oxygen and indocyanine green (93.1).

94 The Mapleson classification originates from a paper discussing rebreathing (94.1).

  a) T When respiring through the 'D' system, the pattern of respiration, to and fro from the expiratory limb, requires that the fresh gas flow must be high enough to wash out the expired gas, a minimum of 3 times minute volume (94.2).

  b) T Because the anatomical dead space gas can take part in the next breath, the 'A' system can use a fresh gas flow equivalent to the alveolar ventilation without a rise in Pa_{CO_2} (94.2).

  c) T The 'B' system has a large dead space in the expiratory limb. It is little used today (94.2).

  d) F The mechanism in any breathing system for matching fresh gas flow with the demand of peak inspiratory flow rate is called the reservoir bag (94.2).

  e) F Both frequency and tidal volume of ventilation make a major contribution to the mechanics of the system (94.2).

95 There continues to be debate about halothane and the liver despite the low incidence of complications attributable to the drug. This is a controversial subject.

Halothane-associated hepatitis:
a) does not occur without previous exposure to halothane
b) has an incidence of about 1 in 10 000 halothane anaesthetics
c) is more common in men
d) occurs more commonly if hypoxia has been present
e) always occurs in the first week after exposure

96 Heparin is given as both prophylaxis and treatment of unwanted clotting. As with any drug it has unwanted effects. Low molecular weight heparins are becoming available.

Heparin:
a) can only be extracted from bovine liver
b) is poorly protein bound
c) enhances the effect of antithrombin III on factor Xa
d) prevents the formation of thrombin from prothrombin
e) thrombocytopenia may occur during treatment

References

95.1	Anaesthesia Review 8	p 179–194

96.1	Dundee, Clarke & McCaughey	p 441
96.2	Souhami & Moxham	p 1104
96.3	Souhami & Moxham	p 1095

95 Halothane associated liver dysfunction may be either mild or severe. The incidence of elevated liver enzyme concentrations in the postoperative period is about 25%. Severe disease is much less common. The exact mechanism is unclear. Direct toxicity is unlikely but there may be either a form of immune sensitisation or a toxic metabolite from an alternate metabolic pathway.

a) F Severe hepatic dysfunction can occur on first exposure but is more likely after subsequent halothane anaesthetics (95.1).

b) F Much less common than this; about 1 in 35 000 or less (95.1).

c) F The sex ratio is F:M, 1.6:1 (95.1).

d) T The hypothesis states that when hypoxia is present a reductive metabolic pathway for halothane predominates, producing a toxic metabolite (95.1).

e) F Hepatitis may occur up to 28 days after exposure (95.1).

96 Heparin is not a pure compound but a biological extract with a wide spectrum of molecular weights.

a) F Heparin, as the name implies, was first extracted from liver but is now commercially extracted from beef lung or pig gut mucosa (96.1).

b) F Heparin is almost totally protein bound (96.1).

c) T Factor Xa converts prothrombin to thrombin and is inhibited by antithrombin III. On exposure to heparin, antithrombin III activity is enhanced (96.2, 96.3).

d) T As described above in c).

e) T Thrombocytopenia seems to be an idiosyncratic reaction rather than a consumptive problem (96.1, 96.2).

97 The monoamine oxidase inhibiting drugs (MAOIs) will be old friends to examination candidates. They are rarely met in modern practice.

In patients taking phenelzine:
a) the effects of phenylephrine will be enhanced
b) the cerebral effects of overdosage may be antagonized by physostigmine
c) pethidine is contraindicated
d) diabetics will require more insulin
e) there is reduced synthesis of cerebral monoamines

98 The metabolic response to surgery is a measurable change in the various biochemical and hormonal factors of catabolism.

The metabolic response to surgery:
a) is delayed but not abolished by high doses of opioids
b) is obtunded by continuous interpleural local anaesthesia
c) is not altered by benzodiazepine premedication
d) features a rise in plasma catecholamines when nitrous oxide is administered
e) is abolished by spinal anaesthesia to T4

References

97.1	Dundee, Clarke & McCaughey	p 563
97.2	Dundee, Clarke & McCaughey	p 359
97.3	BNF	appendix 1
97.4	BNF	section 4.3
98.1	Scurr, Feldman & Soni	p 354–357
98.2	Anaesthesia Review 8	p 127

97 There is still debate as to the exact mechanism of action of MAOIs, but protocols exist for the management of patients taking these drugs. Adrenaline and noradrenaline are both monoamines, hence the incidence of hypertension and problems with similar vasoactive drugs.

   a) F The direct acting vasoconstrictors are not enhanced because noradrenaline is not involved in their mechanism of action. Those drugs with an indirect action will be enhanced. There is still some debate on this point (97.1, 97.2, 97.3, 97.4).

   b) F The hyperexcitability of tricyclic overdose may be treated with physostigmine, but not so the untoward effects of the MAOIs (97.2).

   c) T The response to pethidine, a monoamine, becomes unpredictable in patients on MAOI therapy, giving rise to hyperpyrexia, sweating and hypotension among other effects (97.1).

   d) F The dose requirement for insulin is reduced (97.3).

   e) T The supposed mechanism of action of these drugs is by reduction of the rate of degradation of the catecholamine neurotransmitters. In the long term there is reduced synthesis of cerebral monoamines, presumably by some negative feedback system (97.1).

98 Surgery has metabolic consequences, some detrimental, some advantageous, all poorly understood.

   a) T High doses of opioids delay the response until their offset of action (98.1).

   b) F A new local anaesthetic technique, interpleural anaesthesia does not seem to reduce the metabolic response to surgery (98.2).

   c) F (98.1).

   d) T Nitrous oxide may produce sympathetic stimulation and increased plasma catecholamine levels (98.1).

   e) F The metabolic response to surgery is delayed but not abolished (98.1).

99 The management of most of the common and some of the uncommon poisonings is the province of the anaesthetist. Methanol (methyl alcohol) is readily available and presents some interesting effects on ingestion which are beloved of examiners.

In methanol toxicity:
a) there will be a severe metabolic acidosis
b) ethyl alcohol has a role in treatment
c) methanol will be metabolized to acetaldehyde
d) gluconeogenesis will be inhibited
e) blindness may be a presenting feature

100 **In disseminated intravascular coagulation (DIC):**

a) there will be thrombocytopenia
b) the presence of elevated titres of fibrin degradation products is diagnostic
c) fibrin polymerization is inhibited by fibrin degradation products
d) the prothrombin time will be prolonged
e) the clotting time is reduced

References

99.1   Dundee, Clarke & McCaughey   p 593

100.1 Souhami & Moxham   p 1099

99 Methanol intoxication is rarely severe, largely because the methylated spirit available to the public is unpalatable. The ethanol in the mixture also has some protective effect. Patients present with confusion, ataxia and visual disturbances.

  a) T Methanol inhibits gluconeogenesis and lactate conversion, resulting in a severe metabolic acidosis (99.1).
  b) T Ethanol saturates alcohol dehydrogenase, preventing the oxidation of methanol (99.1).
  c) F Ethanol is metabolized to acetaldehyde, methanol to formaldehyde and formic acid (99.1).
  d) T As above (99.1).
  e) T The formaldehyde and formic acid metabolites of methanol accumulate in the vitreous and optic nerve, causing optic oedema and blindness (99.1).

100 The causes of DIC are legion: pre-eclampsia, amniotic fluid embolus, fetal death-in-utero, placental abruption, fat embolus, septicaemia, massive blood loss, severe head injury, malignant hyperpyrexia and many others. Recognition of the cause and its remedy are the primary aims of treatment, paralleling the need for replacement of blood, platelets and clotting factors. Maintenance of major organ function is imperative due to the massive microvascular fibrin deposition.

  a) T Platelets are consumed along with the other clotting factors (100.1).
  b) F Elevated FDP titres are not diagnostic. Any major surgery or trauma without DIC will cause FDPs to rise (100.1).
  c) T FDPs themselves are a potent antithrombotic, preventing the polymerization of fibrin and the formation of a stable plug (100.1).
  d) T All measures of clotting are prolonged (100.1).
  e) F Despite the apparently misleading title of disseminated intravascular coagulation, the clotting time is prolonged because of the consumption of clotting factors, hence the title (100.1).

101 Patients who suffer from chronic lung disease frequently present for surgory, necessitating knowledge of the clinical features.

In a patient with chronic obstructive pulmonary disease there may be:
a) reduced cardiac dullness
b) finger clubbing
c) a palpable liver edge
d) tracheal tug
e) inspiratory rather than expiratory difficulty

102 The lung has many other functions apart from gas exchange. Metabolism is the most important of these.

The following are metabolized by the lung:
a) acetylcholine
b) angiotensin II
c) propofol
d) bradykinin
e) prostaglandin F

References

101.1	Souhami & Moxham	p 458
101.2	Macleod	p 136
101.3	Souhami & Moxham	p 495
101.4	Nunn	p 59–62
102.1	Souhami & Moxham	p 453
102.2	Guyton	p 211–213
102.3	Miller	p 263
102.4	Vickers, Morgan & Spencer	p 69

101a) T The cardiac outline, as defined by percussion, is less obvious in chronic obstructive pulmonary disease (COPD) because of the intervention of hyperinflated lung (101.1).

b) T Finger clubbing is not a specific sign of anything except chronic inflammation. Patients with COPD may have clubbing, but so will patients suffering from ulcerative colitis, Crohn's disease, bronchiectasis and many other chronic diseases (101.1).

c) T Unless there is severe congestive cardiac failure, the palpable liver edge will not usually be due to hepatic enlargement, but to the hyperinflated lungs pushing down the diaphragm and the liver (101.1).

d) T In COPD the accessory muscles of respiration come into use and diaphragmatic activity is increased. The result is that the trachea is pulled down and the thoracic cage is pulled up on inspiration – a tracheal tug (101.2).

e) F On inspiration, the small airways are held open by the expanding thoracic cage. On expiration these same small airways collapse because of the external pressures applied to them, restricting outward airflow; they behave as Starling resistors (101.1, 101.3, 101.4).

102a) T (102.1).

b) F It is angiotensin I which is converted in the lung to form angiotensin II. This is carried out by angiotensin converting enzyme (ACE), the enzyme blocked by the ACE inhibitor drugs in the management of hypertension (102.1, 102.2).

c) F The fate of propofol remains unclear. 40% appears in urine as the glucuronide, having been metabolized in the liver, but there is a suggestion of pulmonary metabolism. Reference material is limited (102.3, 102.4).

d) T (102.1).

e) T (102.1).

103 The peripheral adrenergic agonists are commonly employed during anaesthesia, often to defray the hypotension associated with subarachnoid and epidural blockade.

Ephedrine:
a) inhibits the breakdown of catecholamines
b) has both direct and indirect activity
c) does not cross the placenta
d) increases uterine vascular resistance in pregnancy
e) dilates the pupil

104 **Arterial pulse pressure may be increased if:**
a) the stroke volume falls
b) the ratio of stroke volume to arterial vascular compliance falls
c) there is an increase in heart rate
d) there is a persistent ductus arteriosus
e) there is aortic valve regurgitation

References

103.1	Synopsis	p 367
103.2	Macintosh	p 138
103.3	Dundee, Clarke & McCaughey	p 359
103.4	Miller	p 489
103.5	Int J Obst Anes (1991) 1	p 3–8
104.1	Guyton	p 159–167

103a) T While not strictly a monoamine oxidase inhibitor, ephedrine does possess this property although it makes only a minor contribution to the vasoconstrictor effect of the drug (103.1,103.2).

b) T Direct activity implies that a drug acts directly on the receptor, while indirect activity suggests that a drug causes the release of a neurotransmitter. Ephedrine does both (103.3, 103.4).

c) F Ephedrine crosses the placenta and may cause fetal tachycardia (103.5).

d) T Uterine vascular resistance is increased by ephedrine, though this effect appears to have no great fetal consequence (103.5).

e) T Structurally, ephedrine is similar to the endogenous catecholamines and so might be expected to dilate the pupil (103.1).

104 The pulse pressure is largely determined by the relationship between stroke volume and vascular compliance. If the stroke volume increases then the pulse pressure increases, but if the compliance increases then the pulse pressure will fall. The pulse pressure is a reflection of how easily the stroke volume is accommodated in the arterial tree.

a) F If the SV falls then the pulse pressure will also fall (104.1).

b) F As above (104.1).

c) F Provided that the cardiac output remains constant, an increase in heart rate will cause a fall in pulse pressure because of the fall in stroke volume (104.1).

d) T In PDA, the diastolic pressure is greatly reduced because of increased run-off from the aorta. The systolic pressure is increased because the excess blood returns to the left side of the heart and so the stroke volume rises (104.1).

e) T The diastolic pressure is low in aortic regurgitation because of increased run-off (to the left ventricle). The systolic pressure is increased because the regurgitated blood is ejected on the next stroke (104.1).

105 Carbon monoxide inhalation is a common method of attempted suicide. It is also one of the causes of death in fires and from poorly ventilated heating systems.

Carbon monoxide:
a) moves the oxyhaemoglobin dissociation curve to the right
b) may cause blistering at toxic concentrations
c) occurs naturally in the human body
d) causes metabolic acidosis
e) may cause hyperpyrexia

106 Examination of the cerebrospinal fluid in viral meningitis will show:
a) turbidity
b) increased lymphocyte count
c) increased glucose concentration
d) increased protein concentration
e) increased lactate concentration

References

105.1 OTM   p 6.54–55
105.2 Souhami & Moxham   p 47

106.1 Macleod   p 240–241
106.2 Souhami & Moxham   p 962
106.3 Davidson   p 833
106.4 OTM   p 21.148–149

105 Carbon monoxide (CO) is poisonous because of its affinity for haemo-globin. This affinity prevents oxygen delivery to the tissues, causing acidosis and hypoxia – despite the pink colour of the patient.

a) F The oxyhaemoglobin dissociation curve is moved to the left, causing increased binding of oxygen to the haemoglobin molecule but preventing release in the periphery (105.1).

b) T Blistering is classically associated with barbiturate poisoning but does occur in other forms of toxicity (105.1, 105.2).

c) T Normal nonsmokers have a blood carbon monoxide concentration of 1–3% derived from the alpha methane carbon atom in the protoporphyrin ring of haemoglobin (105.1).

d) T The metabolic acidosis of CO poisoning results from tissue hypoxia (105.1).

e) T (105.1).

106a) F Turbidity is a function of increased red cell count, which does not occur in viral meningitis (106.3).

b) T But not in bacterial meningitis (106.1, 106.4).

c) F The glucose is usually either low or normal (106.1, 106.2, 106.4).

d) T The protein concentration increases as it does in most inflammatory conditions of the meninges (106.2, 106.4).

e) F The lactate concentration rises in bacterial meningitis (106.4).

107 Systemic vascular resistance will rise with injection of:
 a) enoximone
 b) ephedrine
 c) metaraminol
 d) phenylephrine
 e) isoprenaline

108 Paracetamol overdose is remediable if treated early enough. Note the time qualifier in the stem.

Within 12 hours of overdosage with paracetamol:
 a) there will be increased ventilation
 b) there will be hypothermia
 c) there will be acidosis
 d) treatment with n-acetylcysteine is appropriate
 e) liver damage will be expected if more than 15 g was ingested

References		
107.1 Macintosh		p 138–140
107.2 Dundee, Clarke & McCaughey		p 354
108.1 Souhami & Moxham		p 56–57
108.2 Davidson		p 979

107a) F Enoximone is a phosphodiesterase inhibitor which increases stroke volume, inotropic state and cardiac output while reducing afterload by vasodilatation (107.2).
  b) F Ephedrine appears to cause venoconstriction more than arteriolar constriction so that the SVR does not rise. Cardiac output rises because of increased venous return (107.1, 107.2).
  c) T Metaraminol is a negative chronotrope and positive inotrope with both alpha and beta effects. The SVR rises (107.2).
  d) T Phenylephrine is a close analogue of noradrenaline and is a direct acting arteriolar constrictor (107.2).
  e) F Isoprenaline is a positive inotrope, positive chronotrope and vaso-dilator (107.2).

108 Very little happens within 12 hours of ingestion of excessive doses of paracetamol, except that the stage becomes set for death in hepatic failure a week later. The theory on the toxic effects of paracetamol suggests that it has two metabolic pathways: the oxidative pathway has a high capacity but the reductive pathway produces highly reactive products. In the event of overload of the oxidative pathway (which is limited by glutathione availability), the products of the reductive path-way cause hepatocellular damage. Methionine and acetylcysteine provide glutathione for the oxidative pathway, preventing the accumu-lation of toxic products. Treatment is only effective in the first 12 hours after ingestion. (100.1, 100.2)
  a) F If there is hyperventilation at all in paracetamol overdosage then it will be in the terminal stages rather than in the initial stages (108.1, 108.2).
  b) F There may be a fall in temperature more than 36 hours after ingestion, but not in the first 12 hours (108.2).
  c) F Acidosis only occurs in gross cases and usually after 36 hours (108.1, 108.2).
  d) T See above (108.1, 108.2).
  e) T Significant liver damage has been reported with as little as 15 g ingested (30 standard tablets). The likelihood increases with the quantity ingested (108.1).

109 Fulminant hepatic failure is rare. Unfortunately, the causes are numerous and the treatment difficult.

A patient with fulminant hepatic failure may have:
a) hypokalaemia
b) hypoalbuminaemia
c) an elevated serum bilirubin concentration
d) hypoglycaemia
e) hyperventilation

110 A knowledge of the physiology of obstetric pain pathways is highly desirable. There remains some room for debate on this topic.

The pain of uterine contraction in labour:
a) passes via the nervi erigentes from the cervix
b) passes from the body of the uterus via the lumbar sympathetic chain
c) is perceived in the lower thoracic dermatomes
d) is transmitted via the lower thoracic nerve roots
e) is transmitted from the body of the uterus via the cervical plexus

References

109.1 Davidson   p 511–513
109.2 Souhami & Moxham   p 638–639

110.1 Wall & Melzak   p 484–486

109 Fulminant hepatic failure is defined as acute hepatic failure occurring, within eight weeks of the initiating insult with no obvious pre-existing hepatic dysfunction.

a) T Patients with hepatic failure have secondary hyperaldosteronism, which results in renal potassium loss (109.1, 109.2).

b) F Although patients with chronic hepatic failure will be hypoalbuminaemic because of a failure of production, the patient with fulminant hepatic failure has not had sufficient time for this to become apparent (109.1).

c) T Strangely, the hyperbilirubinaemia of hepatic failure can be both conjugated and unconjugated, depending upon the cause. In cholestatic jaundice, there is an element of obstruction peripheral to the site of conjugation. Either way, hyperbilirubinaemia occurs (109.1).

d) T Hypoglycaemia is one of the two more common causes of death. Glycogen metabolism fails in the ailing liver (109.2).

e) T The acidosis and uraemia of hepatic failure lead to hyperventilation in the terminal stages (109.2).

110 There is confusion over the neuroanatomy of labour pain pathways. The received wisdom is that fibres from the uterine body pass via the lower thoracic nerve roots and that the fibres from the lower segment of uterus and cervix pass via the pudendal nerve to the sacral segments. This is not the whole truth. The fibres from the uterine body pass through the cervical plexus to the lumbar sympathetic chain, up to the lower thoracic chain and then enter the spinal cord via the rami comitantes rather than the nerve root. The cervical fibres are involved in the sympathetic pathways of the pelvis, via the pudendal nerves (110.1). Some discrepancies will be found between references.

a) F (110.1).
b) T See above (110.1).
c) T (110.1).
d) F Via the sympathetics rather than the somatic roots (110.1).
e) T See above (110.1).

111 Splitting of the heart sounds may be a valuable sign of pathology and may be missed on physical examination.

A split second heart sound may be:
a) due to an atrial septal defect
b) normal
c) present in pregnancy
d) present in congestive cardiac failure
e) present in hypertrophic cardiomyopathy

112 Do not be tempted to guess. Only answer for those drugs of which you have certain knowledge.

The following drugs alter the activity of the mixed function oxidase enzymes in the liver:
a) cimetidine
b) rifampicin
c) ketoconazole
d) phenytoin
e) barbiturates

References

111.1 Davidson		p 257–258
111.2 Macleod		p 103–104
112.1 Davidson		p 514

111a) T In atrial septal defect, the blood is shunted from left to right which increases the work of the right side of the heart and delays the pulmonary component of the second sound (111.1, 111.2).

b) T In young persons and on inspiration the venous return to the left side is delayed while the return to the right is increased; this causes a slight difference in the timing of the two components of the second sound (111.1, 111.2).

c) F The added sound most commonly found in pregnancy is the third sound (111.1).

d) F Splitting of the second sound is abolished by cardiac failure (111.2).

e) T Hypertrophic cardiomyopathy causes a delay in ejection from the ventricle and a delay in the closure of the aortic valve – a split sound (111.1, 111.2).

112 Note that the stem says 'alter', not 'increase', 'decrease' or 'induce'.

a) T Cimetidine reduces the activity of these enzymes (112.1).

b) T Activity is increased (112.1).

c) T Activity is reduced (112.1).

d) T Activity is increased (112.1).

e) T Barbiturates are the classic example of drugs which increase the activity of these enzymes (112.1).

113 Questions concerning drug effects upon the pregnant uterus are not restricted to the agents commonly used in clinical obstetric practice for their contracting or relaxing properties.

Uterine contractility in pregnancy:
a) is increased by terbutaline
b) is increased by noradrenaline
c) is reduced by cortisol
d) is reduced by adrenaline
e) is reduced by salbutamol

114 When measuring systemic arterial pressure, falsely high readings may be caused by:
a) the use of too narrow a cuff
b) arteriosclerosis
c) obese arms
d) use of the stethoscope diaphragm
e) too rapid release of pressure in the cuff

References

113.1 Rang & Dale   p 182–185
113.2 Wall & Melzack   p 490

114.1 Macleod   p 91
114.2 Souhami & Moxham   p 437
114.3 Davidson   p 255

113 Contractions of the uterus in pregnancy are intrinsic. The effect on uterine contractility seen with most sympathomimetic drugs depends upon their alpha and beta characteristics. In general, alpha$_1$ stimulation increases uterine tone while beta$_2$ stimulation causes relaxation. Drugs which have both beta$_1$ and beta$_2$ agonist effects will reveal their beta$_2$ effect on the uterus and bronchi, and their beta$_1$ effects on the cardiovascular system.

a) F Terbutaline is a beta$_2$ agonist usually used as a bronchodilator (113.1).

b) T Noradrenaline has pure alpha agonist effects and so causes an increase in uterine tone. This is uncoordinated so is of no therapeutic value (113.1).

c) T (113.2).

d) T Adrenaline has predominantly beta agonist actions and so reduces uterine tone. There is a rebound increase in tone after the infusion is stopped (113.1).

e) T Salbutamol is a beta agonist with mixed beta$_1$ and beta$_2$ effects. The beta$_2$ effects cause uterine relaxation, for which it has been used therapeutically, while the beta$_1$ effects limit this use because of tachycardia (113.1).

114 Systemic arterial pressure is surprisingly variable. It is very difficult to obtain accurate and consistent results. Even intra-arterial monitoring may give inaccurate results if set up incorrectly (measurement of the frequency response and damping of the system are of great importance).

a) T If the cuff is too narrow then the pressure required to occlude the artery will be higher (114.1, 114.2, 114.3).

b) T The 'blood pressure' is really the pressure inside the artery. The resistance to occlusion of the vessel wall is another matter. It is the resistance to occlusion which is increased in arteriosclerosis, giving a falsely high reading (114.3).

c) T Obese arms cause the same problem as arteriosclerosis, increased resistance to occlusion (114.1).

d) F The diaphragm tends to pick up higher frequency sound than the bell. This is of little relevance.

e) F If the cuff pressure is released too quickly then the pressure recorded will tend to be inaccurately low because of the delay between passing the true pressure and the visualization of the reading (114.1).

115 Adult pyloric stenosis is less frequently encountered than its juvenile counterpart. There are some shared biochemical features.

The following results are compatible with a diagnosis of adult pyloric stenosis:
a) serum chloride 106 mmol/l
b) serum sodium 127 mmol/l
c) serum urea 18 mmol/l
d) serum bicarbonate 40 mmol/l
e) serum potassium 6 mmol/l

116 A second question on tetanus which has a different emphasis to its predecessor. Compare Question 54.

Tetanus:
a) does not present in infancy
b) can be prevented by antibiotics
c) presents with dysphagia early in the disease
d) may present with ocular involvement
e) causes sympathetic paralysis

References
115.1 Dunnill & Colvin   p 71–76
115.2 Zilva & Pannall   p 97–98

116.1 Davidson   p 885–886
116.2 Stoelting   p 652–653

115 Adult pyloric stenosis is no longer common since the introduction of H_2 receptor blockers. When it does occur there is loss of chloride and hydrogen ion from the stomach during vomiting, which is not balanced by loss of bicarbonate and sodium from the duodenum. The result is a hypochloraemic alkalosis with poor renal compensation, almost always accompanied by hypokalaemia. Normal serum values in mmol/l are: chloride 95–105, sodium 135–148, urea 2.5–6.5, bicarbonate 24–32, potassium 3.8–5 (115.1).

   a) F The serum chloride concentration will be low because of loss from the stomach (115.2).

   b) F Dehydration and continued production by the gastric parietal cells will increase the serum sodium concentration (115.2).

   c) T Dehydration will tend to increase the serum urea concentration (115.2).

   d) T The serum bicarbonate concentration will rise because of continued gastric cell production which is not matched by renal loss (115.2).

   e) F Hypochloraemic alkalosis is almost always accompanied by hypokalaemia (115.2). See above.

116 Prevention and reduction of mortality from tetanus depends upon immunization schedules and intensive care facilities which may not always be available.

   a) F Neonatal tetanus is a major problem in the third world and would respond to improved conditions in the place of delivery (116.1).

   b) T Large doses of simple antibiotics soon after injury can prevent the multiplication of the causal organism, *Clostridium tetani* (116.1).

   c) F Trismus is more common as a presenting feature than dysphagia (116.1).

   d) F Risus sardonicus, the fixed stare of facial muscle spasm in tetanus, is not an eye sign but a sign of generalized facial spasm (116.1).

   e) F In tetanus there are sympathetic 'storms' which may prove fatal despite heavy sedation and ventilation. Sympathetic paralysis is not an accepted term for this event (116.2).

117 Understanding of the importance of ventilation and perfusion distribution is central to respiratory physiology.

An area of lung with a decreased ventilation/perfusion ratio:
a) is an area of shunt
b) is an area of physiological dead space
c) is responsible for a fall in Pa_{O_2} without a change in Pa_{CO_2}
d) will show hypoxic vasoconstriction
e) may be compensated for by increasing ventilation

118 **The following are true of methods of oxygen analysis:**
a) a paramagnetic analyser measures the percentage of oxygen in the analysed gas
b) a mass spectrometer is rendered inaccurate by the presence of nitrous oxide
c) infrared absorption can be used for breath-by-breath analysis
d) the Haldane method is inaccurate in the presence of nitrous oxide
e) the polarographic method consumes oxygen

References

117.1	West	p 51–68
117.2	West	p 17–19
117.3	Nunn	p 127–128
118.1	Scurr, Feldman & Soni	p 116–117
118.2	Churchill–Davidson	p 141–142

117 A decreased ventilation/perfusion ratio implies either that the ventilation to a segment of lung has been reduced without a parallel reduction in perfusion, or that the perfusion has been increased without a parallel rise in ventilation.

a) F Shunt is the passage of venous blood to the left side of the heart without passing through a ventilated area of lung. There is a V/Q ratio of zero (117.1).

b) F Physiological dead space is a measure of the volume of lung which is not involved in carbon dioxide exchange. Physiological dead space has an infinite V/Q ratio (117.2).

c) T The pulmonary arterial blood does not unload as much oxygen as usual in this situation and behaves like a shunt (but is not true shunt), reducing the Pa_{O_2} without increasing the Pa_{CO_2} (117.1).

d) T A decrease in ventilation will cause the onset of hypoxic vaso-constriction, thus limiting shunting (117.3).

e) T Only true if the increased ventilation is to that section of lung. If the problem is one of a regional reduction in compliance, the increased ventilation may go to a more compliant section of lung (117.1).

118 Here is a catch for the unwary. The stem clearly states 'oxygen analysis'.

a) F Paramagnetic analysers measure partial pressure, not percentage (118.1).

b) F The mass spectrometer depends upon the mass/charge ratio of ions in a specimen of gas after bombardment by electrons. Gases which have the same molecular weight give superimposed peaks and so cause confusion. The gases used in anaesthesia which do this are carbon dioxide and nitrous oxide, both having a molecular weight of 44. The measurement of oxygen is not affected (118.1).

c) F Infrared absorption is not a method used for oxygen analysis (118.1).

d) F The Haldane method relies upon the absorption of carbon dioxide by potassium hydroxide. This causes a measurable fall in the volume of the sample. The oxygen in the sample is then absorbed by pyrogallol, leaving a residual volume of other gases. Potassium hydroxide also absorbs nitrous oxide and, therefore, if carbon dioxide is the gas being measured, there will be an inaccuracy in the volume remaining. However, it is the oxygen which is being measured and thus there is no inaccuracy (118.2).

e) T The polarographic electrode depends upon the electrical current produced in an electrolyte solution between two charged plates when oxygen is reduced (118.2).

119 Drugs which affect renal function and therefore electrolyte balance may have considerable impact upon anaesthetic management. Diuretic agents are widely prescribed.

The loop diuretics may cause:
a) hyponatraemia
b) hypokalaemic alkalosis
c) hypochloraemia
d) hyperuricaemia
e) hypermagnesaemia

120 The clinical features of pulmonary embolism may be extrapolated from a knowledge of the pathological process.

Features of pulmonary thromboembolism may include:
a) elevated Pa_{CO_2}
b) reduced Pa_{O_2}
c) bronchospasm
d) increased surfactant activity
e) reduced ventilation/perfusion ratio

References

119.1	Rang & Dale	p 319–323
119.2	Zilva & Pannall	p 65–66
119.3	Zilva & Pannall	p 381–383
120.1	Nunn	p 448–449
120.2	Souhami & Moxham	p 502–503

119 The loop diuretics include frusemide, bumetanide and ethacrinic acid.

a) T The loop diuretics inhibit tubular reabsorption of sodium and chloride, causing hyponatraemia in addition to the other effects discussed below (119.1).

b) T Loop diuretics cause an increased sodium load to be delivered to the distal tubule, where sodium is exchanged for both potassium and hydrogen ion. The net effect is to increase bicarbonate reabsorption which, combined with the potassium loss, presents as hypokalaemic alkalosis (119.1, 119.2).

c) T Chloride is lost along with sodium (119.1).

d) F The thiazides reduce tubular excretion of uric acid. The loop diuretics do not (119.3).

e) F The loop diuretics cause urinary loss of magnesium and calcium (119.1).

120 The physiological upset of non-lethal pulmonary embolus can be considerable and longstanding. Lung architecture is arranged to mini-mize the damage of embolism and to repair that damage as rapidly as possible. The initial effect is of an increase in alveolar dead space which is later compensated for by bronchospasm and reduced ventilation.

a) F The Pa_{CO_2} is usually reduced by hyperventilation rather than elevated by the shunt (120.1).

b) T The diversion of blood away from ventilated alveoli will cause the arterial P_{O_2} to fall by venous admixture (120.1).

c) T The local release of serotonin by platelets involved in the intravas-cular clotting process causes bronchospasm in the affected area (120.1).

d) F Note that the two references cited differ slightly. While (120.1) gives the impression that the amount of surfactant is normal but is opposed by fibrin from the clot, (120.2) suggests the amount of surfactant is reduced (120.1, 120.2).

e) F An increase in alveolar dead space, i.e. a reduction in perfusion relative to ventilation, is an increase in ventilation/perfusion ratio, not a reduction (120.1).

121 Glycosuria is commonly found in diabetes mellitus but there are other causes. Remember that the tubular maxima for glucose demonstrate a splay in absolute values.

Glycosuria may occur in:
a) normal pregnancy
b) post gastrectomy patients
c) hypopituitarism
d) patients taking loop diuretics
e) hypothyroidism

122 The alkaline phosphatases are a group of enzymes which hydrolyse phosphates at high pH. There are several isoenzymes of this group formed in bone, liver, intestine and placenta.

Elevated levels of alkaline phosphatase may be found in:
a) myelomatosis
b) pregnancy
c) cholestasis
d) Paget's disease of bone
e) osteoporosis

References

121.1	Davidson	p 666–667
121.2	Davidson	p 614–617
121.3	Zilva & Pannall	p 210–211
122.1	Davidson	p 493–494
122.2	Zilva & Pannall	p 146–147
122.3	Zilva & Pannall	p 304–306
122.4	Zilva & Pannall	p 183–188

121 Glycosuria may be the result of increased glucose load on the kidney or reduced renal reabsorption. In young people it may be normal because of a lower renal threshold.

a) T In pregnancy the renal threshold for glucose falls, allowing glycosuria to occur. This must be distinguished from 'gestational diabetes' where the patient behaves as a diabetic but only during, or just after, pregnancy (121.1).

b) T After extensive gastric surgery, a glucose load may be presented to the small bowel and absorbed rapidly, giving a high peak which exceeds the renal threshold. This contrasts with the normal pattern of gastric absorption, in which blood glucose does not reach such high levels (121.1).

c) F Patients with reduced pituitary function tend towards hypoglycaemia and therefore glycosuria is unlikely to occur (121.2).

d) F Thiazide diuretics tend to cause glycosuria rather than the loop diuretics (121.3).

e) F Glycosuria tends to occur in hyper- rather than hypothyroid states (121.1).

122a) F Myeloma is not usually associated with increased bone deposition and so the alkaline phosphatase is not raised (122.1).

b) T The placenta in normal pregnancy is a major source of alkaline phosphatase (122.1, 122.2).

c) T In cholestatic jaundice, the alkaline phosphatase manufactured by the hepatic cells is released into the circulation because of the obstruction. This provides a very sensitive index of hepatocellular damage (122.3).

d) T In Paget's disease of bone, there is increased osteoblastic activity and bone deposition (unlike myeloma). The alkaline phosphatase is released from osteoblasts in line with their increased activity (122.4).

e) F In osteomalacia, increased osteoblastic activity is accompanied by poor calcium availability, bone is softened and the alkaline phosphatase is high. In osteoporosis there is no increased osteoblast activity and no increase in alkaline phosphatase (122.4).

123 Myoglobin is a constituent of striated muscle. Myoglobinuria results from breakdown of muscle, and in large quantities it can cause significant renal damage.

Myoglobinuria may be associated with:
a) severe exercise
b) an inborn error of metabolism
c) a positive urine test for blood
d) elevated blood levels of creatine kinase
e) reduced blood calcium concentration

124 Mitral valve stenosis may be met in the clinical part of the examination.

Each of the following intracardiac pressure measurements might be found in a patient with severe mitral stenosis:
a) pulmonary artery pressure 20/10 mmHg
b) right ventricular pressure 20/3 mmHg
c) left venticular pressure 110/5 mmHg
d) pulmonary artery wedge pressure 10 mmHg
e) left atrial pressure 5 mmHg

References

123.1 OTM   p 26.6–7

124.1 Macleod   p 119
124.2 Davidson   p 294

123 Myoglobin is usually identifiable in plasma in low concentration. High concentrations may be found after severe metabolic or physical muscle insult, including severe exercise. In high concentrations, the renal glomeruli may become obstructed and renal failure ensues.

a) **T** Marathon running is the classical exercise-induced cause of myoglobinuria (123.1).

b) **T** Carnitine palmityl transferase deficiency, with which we are doubtless well acquainted, causes congenital moderate myoglobinuria (123.1).

c) **T** Stick tests for blood are not specific enough to separate myoglobin from haemoglobin (123.1).

d) **T** Muscle damage and high turnover of muscle protein elevate plasma creatine kinase (123.1).

e) **T** Damaged muscle takes up calcium from the blood, and hypocalcaemia is an almost universal finding in myoglobinuria (123.1).

124 All the cited pressures are <u>normal</u>. In severe mitral stenosis only the left ventricular pressure might be normal, while the other pressures tend to be raised (124.1, 124.2).

a) **F**
b) **F**
c) **T**
d) **F**
e) **F**

125 The investigation of jaundiced patients must include a detailed drug history, based upon the knowledge of the extensive list of drugs known to cause jaundice.

The following drugs may cause jaundice:
a) ranitidine
b) metronidazole
c) cimetidine
d) chlorpropamide
e) erythromicin

126 The consequences of the more common malignancies are not merely local to the tumour but may have a range of far reaching effects. Carcinoma of the prostate is a common malignancy.

In carcinoma of the prostate:
a) it almost always presents with retention of urine
b) the bone secondaries are osteolytic rather than osteosclerotic
c) the plasma alkaline phosphatase is usually elevated
d) oestrogens may be used in the management
e) it is often only diagnosed after prostatic resection

References

125.1	Goodman & Gilman	p 900–901
125.2	Goodman & Gilman	p 1004–1005
125.3	Souhami & Moxham	p 636–637
125.4	Goodman & Gilman	p 1132–1133
126.1	Davidson	p 604–605
126.2	Stoelting	p 685

125 It is difficult to say with assurance that a particular drug will <u>not</u> cause jaundice, much more difficult than to say it <u>does</u>. The references to the false completions below do not mention jaundice as an unwanted effect.
  a) F (125.1).
  b) F (125.2).
  o) T (125.1).
  d) T (125.3).
  e) T (125.3, 125.4).

126a) F Carcinoma of prostate may present with urine retention but more usually presents with secondary effects, such as backache from spinal metastases or anaemia (126.1).
  b) F The bony lesions of metastatic prostatic cancer are sclerotic rather than lytic (126.2).
  c) F Although the alkaline phosphatase may be elevated in prostatic cancer, it is the <u>acid</u> phosphatase which is the marker of the tumour (126.1).
  d) T Stilboestrol and other oestrogenic drugs may be used in prostatic cancer, the purpose being to deprive the tumour of androgenic support. There is some doubt about the effectiveness of hormonal manipulation. It may make the patient feel better, but the effect on survival is not yet clear (126.1). Bilateral orchidectomy may be the treatment of choice.
  e) T Prostatic cancer is frequently diagnosed on histology of resection specimens without prior suspicion (126.1).

127 A number of patients presenting for surgery are overweight. The definition of morbid obeslty may be taken as body weight greater than twice ideal.

In the obese patient:
a) the functional residual capacity is reduced
b) left ventricular failure is common
c) there is an increased incidence of thromboembolism
d) more fluoride ion is produced from enflurane than in the non-obese
e) intragastric pH and volume are increased

128 Anorexia nervosa is associated with:
a) diabetes insipidus
b) shortening of the Q–T interval
c) acidosis
d) hyperkalaemia
e) hypercalcaemia

References

127.1	Miller	p 801–802
128.1	Miller	p 802
128.2	Stoelting	p 546–567

127 The physiological changes of obesity are complex. Although fat is a vessel-poor tissue, the sheer mass of it makes it effectively vessel-rich and so a higher proportion of the cardiac output is diverted there. The weight of fat on the chest reduces FRC even when the patient is awake, and increases the intra-abdominal pressure.
   a) T (127.1).
   b) F In general, obese patients develop right heart failure (127.1).
   c) T Because of the increase in intra-abdominal pressure and the weight of fat on the legs, the peripheral venous return is sluggish and the patients are more prone to thromboembolism (127.1).
   d) T Explanation is lacking here. Presumably the absorption of enflurane into the increased fat depot means that the drug is exposed to metabolism for longer and so is metabolized more extensively than in the non-obese (127.1).
   e) F Read the question! Although intragastric volume rises, pH falls. The completion suggests that the contents would be more alkaline than normal whereas they are in fact more acid (127.1).

128 Anorexia nervosa and starvation have much in common. They are both conditions of gross protein, caloric and fat deprivation.
   a) T Patients with anorexia nervosa develop a condition similar to panhypopituitarism in that they cannot control their body temperature, sexual characteristics (such as menses) and they cannot concentrate urine (128.1, 128.2).
   b) F The Q–T interval is often prolonged in anorexia nervosa (128.1).
   c) T The metabolic burning of fat and protein rather than glucose produces organic acids from the Krebs and fatty acid cycles, which cannot be metabolized further without glucose (128.1).
   d) F Hypokalaemia is more usual than hyperkalaemia (128.1).
   e) F Hypocalcaemia is more common (128.1).

129 The inhibition of platelet aggregation by a drug may be desirable or undesirable. Both features are represented in the completions below.

Aggregation of platelets is inhibited by:
a) aminocaproic acid
b) disopyramide
c) heparin
d) sulphinpyrazone
e) dipyridamole

130 Hypothermia is met as a consequence of drug ingestion and disease process. The anaesthetized patient is rendered poikilothermic.

Accidental hypothermia may be associated with:
a) hypocapnia
b) chlorpromazine
c) pancreatitis
d) aspirin poisoning
e) reduced skeletal muscle tone

References

129.1	Goodman & Gilman	p 1325–1326
129.2	Goodman & Gilman	p 848–857
129.3	Goodman & Gilman	p 1313–1317
129.4	Goodman & Gilman	p 746–747
130.1	Souhami & Moxham	p 78–79
130.2	Davidson	p 979
130.3	Davidson	p 85–86
130.4	Souhami & Moxham	p 54–55

129a) F Aminocaproic acid stimulates coagulation. It appears to have no effect upon platelets (129.1).

b) F Disopyramide and dipyridamole (see **e**) are names which are easily confused. Disopyramide is an antiarrhythmic agent with no platelet effect (129.2).

c) T Heparin in ordinary doses has no effect on platelets but in large doses causes reduced platelet aggregation (129.3).

d) T Sulphinpyrazone is a derivative of phenylbutazone with a uricosuric action. It is also used as an antiplatelet agent (129.1, 129.4).

e) T Dipyridamole is a specific inhibitor of platelet aggregation. It is not as effective as aspirin but may be used if there is a history of peptic ulceration or aspirin allergy (129.1).

130 Note that the stem states 'is associated with' rather than 'causes' or 'is caused by'.

a) F The respiratory depression that occurs in hypothermia tends to cause hypercapnia (130.1).

b) T Chlorpromazine is notorious for preventing shivering. It is also a potent alpha adrenergic blocker and as such can cause significant hypothermia by vasidilatation (130.1, 130.2).

c) T Hypothermia of any duration may cause pancreatitis, although it is uncommon (130.3).

d) F Aspirin may cause hypothermia by uncoupling oxidative phosphorylation (130.4).

e) F Patients with hypothermia tend to have high resting muscle tone (130.1).

131 Know the list of drugs to avoid and the drugs which are safe to use in the various porphyric states.

The following drugs should be avoided in acute intermittent porphyria (AIP):
a) diclofenac
b) droperidol
c) etomidate
d) phenytoin
e) propofol

132 Starch solutions are becoming available for the treatment of hypovolaemia. Some aspects of treatment with these solutions have not yet been fully resolved.

Solutions of hydroxyethyl starch (hetastarch, pentastarch):
a) have a similar average molecular weight to albumin
b) do not affect the haemostatic mechanisms
c) are eliminated via the kidney
d) are taken up into the reticuloendothelial system
e) cause an increase in plasma volume more than the infused volume

References		
131.1 BNF	section 10.1	
131.2 Stoelting	p 529–532	
131.3 Miller	p 847–848	
131.4 Anaesthesia Review 6	p 303–304	
131.5 BJA (1992) 68:2	p 230	
132.1 Zilva & Pannall	p 328	
132.2 Miller	p 1459	
132.3 Miller	p 1495–1496	

131a) I But note that references to diclofenac in the 'safe' or 'avoid' categories are infrequent (131.1).
 b) F Droperidol seems to be safe to use in AIP (131.2, 131.3).
 c) T Stoelting (131.2) suggests that etomidate is to be avoided, while Miller (131.3) suggests that it is safe. Perhaps the best answer would therefore be to avoid the completion.
 d) T Phenytoin should be avoided (131.2, 131.3).
 e) F There is limited experience with propofol in porphyria but that which exists suggests that it is not unsafe (131.4). A recent case report substantiates this view (131.5).

132 Starch solutions are solutions of synthetic polysaccharides which, being non-biological in origin, avoid the infective and reactive problems of other solutions.
 a) F The average molecular weight of the starch solutions is 450 000 daltons. That of albumin is 65 000 daltons (132.1, 132.2, 132.3).
 b) F At doses above 1000 ml/70 kg, factor VIII is reduced (132.3).
 c) T The smaller molecular weight fragments of starch are eliminated quickly by the kidney. The larger fragments are metabolized over a longer period before being eliminated in bile and urine (132.2).
 d) T The starch molecules are taken up into the reticuloendothelial system of the liver before elimination over a prolonged period of time (132.3).
 e) T Volume replacement and plasma expansion are often used as synonyms but there is a difference. Volume replacement implies that the circulating volume is increased by the transfused volume, whereas plasma expansion implies that the circulating volume is increased by more than the infused volume, usually because water is drawn in from the tissues by the infused solution. The starch solutions, because of their high molecular weight, act as expanders rather than replacers (132.3).

133 Thrombosis and embolism are common causes of morbidity and mortality. The aetiology and prevention of deep venous thrombosis (DVT) are common examination topics.

The incidence of deep venous thrombosis is increased in the presence of:
a) malignant disease
b) high cardiac output states
c) pregnancy
d) cardiac failure
e) ulcerative colitis

134 In a patient diagnosed as having an extradural haematoma causing spinal cord compression:
a) the patient may have leukaemia
b) there may be an arterio-venous malformation in the epidural space
c) lack of bladder symptoms may cause the diagnosis to be reviewed
d) there will probably be a clotting disorder
e) the diagnosis can only be made radiologically

References

133.1	Davidson	p 338–339
133.2	Souhami & Moxham	p 449
133.3	Moir	p 347
134.1	Anaesthesia (1985) 40	p 1219–1225
134.2	Souhami & Moxham	p 926–931

133 The incidence of DVT is increased in any state of hypercoagulability, immobility and venous stasis, especially following pelvic or lower limb surgery and during bedrest with limited mobility.
  a) T Precisely which malignancies predispose to DVT is not clear (133.1).
  b) F Low cardiac output states predispose to DVT, presumably because of the sluggish blood flow (133.1).
  c) T The blood of pregnant women is hypercoagulable (133.3).
  d) T As above, presumably because of the sluggish circulation, there is a higher incidence of DVT (133.2).
  e) T DVT is one of the many complications of ulcerative colitis (133.1).

134 Acute paraplegia from iatrogenic epidural haematoma is one of the great fears of every anaesthetist. The anaesthetist may not be at fault, because there is an incidence of spontaneous epidural haematoma. The incidence of haematoma after labour epidural is extremely low (134.1).
  a) T Patients with leukaemia have a tendency to spontaneous haemorrhage (134.2).
  b) T Arterio-venous malformation is not unknown as a cause of paraplegia and cord compression (134.2).
  c) F Back pain and progressive weakness of the lower limbs should suggest cord compression, whether or not the bladder is involved. If the bladder is involved the situation is urgent (134.2).
  d) F Spontaneous haematoma may occur without a clotting defect being detectable (134.2).
  e) F The diagnosis must be suspected if there is weakness and back pain. It can be confirmed by radiological investigations, myelogram or CT scan for example (134.2).

135 Questions on local anaesthetic agents will be met in every part of the anaesthetic diploma examination. Bupivacaine remains the most popular member of this group. The formulation referred to here is Marcain®. Other formulations may differ.

Bupivacaine:
a) is an amide local anaesthetic
b) increases the speed of cardiac conduction
c) may be used in 0.25% solution for intravenous regional anaesthesia (IVRA)
d) the hyperbaric solution for spinal anaesthesia contains 60 mg/ml of dextrose
e) the 0.5% solution contains bupivacaine at a concentration of 50 mg/ml

136 Consider the stem carefully. The causes of unilateral and bilateral pleural effusions are not identical.

Unilateral pleural effusion may be associated with:
a) pulmonary embolism
b) asbestos
c) ovarian fibroma
d) nephrotic syndrome
e) myxoedema

References

135.1	Goodman & Gilman	p 311–330
135.2	Data Sheet Compendium	p 104
136.1	Davidson	p 408–413
136.2	Souhami & Moxham	p 530–534
136.3	Souhami & Moxham	p 694–695

135a) T The majority of local anaesthetic agents used today are amides (135.1).
  b) F Bupivacaine slows cardiac conduction and depresses myocardial contractility (135.1).
  c) F Because of its adverse cardiac effects, bupivacaine is contraindicated in IVRA (135.1).
  d) F 'Heavy Marcain'® is 5.28 mg/ml of bupivacaine hydrochloride in dextrose monohydrate 80 mg/ml (8%) which has a specific gravity of 1026 at 20°C (135.2).
  e) F The true concentration is 5.28 mg/ml, not 60 mg/ml as in this question. This information is written on the ampoule (135.2).

136 Pleural effusion may be difficult to diagnose clinically but may more often be found radiologically. The type of effusion – chylous, serous, blood stained or purulent – can only be assessed by aspiration.
  a) T Pulmonary embolism and infarction can cause effusion of the opposite side! (136.1, 136.2).
  b) T Asbestos inhalation causes mesothelioma, pulmonary fibrosis and benign pleural effusion (136.1).
  c) T This is Meigs' syndrome: ovarian tumour, (not necessarily malignant) ascites and pleural effusion. The effusion resolves with removal of the tumour (136.2).
  d) T Nephrotic syndrome appears to cause pleural effusion because of hypoproteinaemia (136.1).
  e) T Fluid may accumulate in any serous cavity in myxoedema (including the pleural cavity) (136.3).

137 The following are true of the nerve supply to the larynx:
a) the recurrent laryngeal nerve supplies the mucous membrane below the true vocal cords
b) the internal laryngeal nerve supplies the mucous membrane above the true vocal cords
c) the recurrent laryngeal nerve supplies the cricothyroid muscle
d) the external laryngeal nerve is entirely sensory
e) the larynx has no sympathetic nerve supply

138 Be prepared to be handed any of the following examples of double lumen endobronchial tubes in the viva section of the examination.

Of the various types of double lumen endobronchial tube:
a) the Carlen's tube is available in both left- and right-sided versions
b) the Broncho-cath® has a carinal hook
c) the lumen of a Robertshaw tube has a circular cross-section
d) the left-sided Robertshaw tube has a carinal hook
e) the position of the left upper lobe bronchus makes it necessary to have a slot in the bronchial portion of the tube

References	
137.1 Gray	p 1258–1259
137.2 Gray	p 1116–1117
138.1 Churchill-Davidson	p 382–385
138.2 Kaplan	p 371–387

137a) T (137.1).
   b) T (137.1).
   c) F The recurrent laryngeal nerve supplies all the intrinsic muscles of the larynx <u>except</u> the cricothyroid (137.1).
   d) F The external laryngeal nerve is mainly sensory but also supplies the cricothyroid muscle (see above) (137.1).
   e) F The sympathetic supply to the larynx is from the superior cervical ganglion via the superior and then internal laryngeal nerves (137.2).

138a) F The Carlen's tube is always left-sided. There is a similar right-sided tube but it bears the name of White (138.1, 138.2).
   b) F The Broncho-cath® is basically a plastic Robertshaw tube and has no carinal hook (138.1, 138.2).
   c) F The lumen of a Robertshaw tube is D-shaped and the overall profile is oval, resulting in maximum luminal area for gas flow and suctioning (138.1, 138.2).
   d) F Neither right nor left Robertshaw tubes have a carinal hook (138.1, 138.2).
   e) F It is the position of the <u>right</u> upper lobe bronchus which necessitates the slotted bronchial portion in <u>right</u> sided tubes. The left upper lobe bronchus arises further down the main bronchus, away from the tip of an endobronchial tube (138.1, 138.2).

139 Parkinson's disease is a disorder of dopaminergic transmission in the basal ganglia. Features include tremor, difficulty in initiating movement and expressionless facies.

Parkinson's disease:
a) features lead-pipe type rigidity in the legs
b) may be a late complication of carbon monoxide poisoning
c) results in a tremor which is accentuated by movement
d) affects the patient's requirement for muscle relaxant drugs
e) causes dry skin

140 Prior to sitting this examination, seek the help of the radiology department with particular reference to the interpretation of the chest radiograph.

On a PA chest X-ray, the trachea could be deviated to the left:
a) if there were a left pneumothorax
b) if there were left lower lobe pneumonia
c) if there were a left pleural effusion
d) if there were a left phrenic nerve paralysis
e) if the patient were rotated to the left

References

139.1	Davidson	p 868–871
139.2	Stoelting	p 304–306
140.1	Davidson	p 347
140.2	Davidson	p 388–391
140.3	Souhami & Moxham	p 461–464

139a) T The rigidity of this condition is said to be 'cogwheel' in nature. While this may be so in the arms, in the trunk and legs there is more 'lead-pipe' type rigidity (139.1).
  b) T The basal ganglia may be damaged by hypoxia, including that seen in carbon monoxide poisoning (139.2).
  c) F The tremor of Parkinson's disease is reduced by movement, rather than accentuated (139.1, 139.2).
  d) F The dose requirement for muscle relaxants drugs is unchanged, but the dose requirement for cholinergic and anticholinergic drugs is increased (139.2).
  e) F Patients with Parkinson's disease tend to have greasy rather than dry skin (139.1, 139.2).

140 The trachea may be pushed or pulled from its central position by lesions which increase or decrease the volume of a hemithorax.
  a) F In pneumothorax, the intrapleural pressure of the unaffected side is not balanced by that of the affected side and therefore the trachea and mediastinum shift away from the affected side in simple, tension and open pneumothoraces. In tension pneumothorax there is an increase in volume of the affected side (140.1).
  b) T There is a loss of lung volume on the affected side and the trachea is pulled toward that side (140.1, 140.2).
  c) F Pleural effusion does little to change the volume of a hemithorax, unless it pushes the mediastinal structures to the opposite side (140.1), a feature of large volume effusion.
  d) F Phrenic nerve palsy and other conditions affecting motility of the hemidiaphragms cause elevation of the diaphragm on that side with a compensatory loss of lung volume. The volume of the hemithorax is unchanged and so the trachea tends to remain central (140.3).
  e) T The trachea is an anterior structure in the midline of the mediastinum. Thus, if the patient is rotated to the left, the trachea will also appear to be displaced to the left on both AP and PA films (140.3).

141 Anaesthetic gases are usually supplied in cylinders. Oxygen is supplied to larger consumers as a liquid. Modern cylinders are made of molybdenum steel.

In anaesthetic gas cylinders:
a) the filling ratio of a nitrous oxide cylinder is the ratio of the weight of liquid nitrous oxide in the cylinder to the maximum weight of liquid nitrous oxide that it could contain
b) a carbon dioxide cylinder is filled to a pressure of 49 atmospheres
c) the tare weight is the weight of the cylinder when empty
d) a cylinder top which is painted black and white in quarters contains air
e) the valve block is lubricated with a special non-inflammable grease

142 Paroxysmal supraventricular tachycardia:
a) may be terminated by carotid sinus massage
b) may occur in hypothyroidism
c) may be terminated by digoxin
d) may be precipitated by digoxin
e) may respond to verapamil

References

141.1	Ward	p 32–36
142.1	Davidson	p 268–269
142.2	Souhami & Moxham	p 366–369

141a) F The filling ratio of a nitrous oxide cylinder is the ratio of the weight of liquid in the cylinder after filling, to the maximum weight of <u>water</u> which the cylinder could hold (141.1).
b) T (141.1).
c) T (141.1).
d) T (141.1).
e) F The design of valve blocks obviates the need for any kind of lubricant. The behaviour of oils and greases is unpredictable at the high pressures involved and has been the cause of explosions (141.1).

142 The management of supraventricular tachycardia (SVT) falls into distinct phases: recognition, causation, immediate treatment and longer term treatment.
a) T The carotid sinus contains nerve fibres which synapse with the vagus. Stimulation of the carotid sinus causes vagal slowing of the heart which may be enough to terminate an attack of SVT. Pressure on the eyeball may achieve the same end (142.1).
b) F It is hyperthyroid states that predispose to SVT (142.1).
c) T Atrial fibrillation at high ventricular rates is a form of SVT which may be slowed by digoxin therapy (142.1).
d) T SVT is one of the variety of arrhythmias associated with digoxin toxicity (142.2).
e) T Verapamil is the drug of first choice for the termination of an attack of SVT (142.1).

143 Aortic stenosis is a clinical result of several differing pathologies. The net result presents a problem when considering suitable techniques for anaesthesia.

Aortic valvular stenosis may be caused by:
a) congenital bicuspid valve
b) rheumatic fever
c) subacute bacterial endocarditis (SBE)
d) calcified valve cusps
e) ruptured valve cusps

144 Neonatal respiratory distress syndrome:
a) is confined to preterm infants
b) is associated with persistent fetal circulation
c) causes a metabolic acidosis
d) may be associated with pneumomediastinum
e) when the inspired oxygen fraction is too high then there is a risk of retrolental fibroplasia

---

References

143.1	Souhami & Moxham	p 382–384
143.2	Davidson	p 296–303
144.1	Black	p 241–250

143 Patients with aortic stenosis are notorious for developing syncope, intractable arrhythmias and death.
  a) T A significant minority of the population have bicuspid aortic valves which may never cause symptoms. If symptoms develop, valve replacement may become necessary. The functional effect is usually stenosis rather than regurgitation (143.1, 143.2).
  b) T Rheumatic fever can cause stenosis and/or regurgitation in any cardiac valve (143.1, 143.2).
  c) F SBE affects an already damaged valve, and is usually the cause of regurgitation (143.2).
  d) T The calcification may be rheumatic or atherosclerotic (143.1, 143.2).
  e) F Rupture of mitral valve cusps may be the result of ischaemia of the cordae tendinae, but will result in regurgitation. The aortic valve has no such support. Rupture of an aortic cusp results in regurgitation not stenosis (143.2).

144 Neonatal respiratory distress syndrome, also known as hyaline membrane disease, is a condition of preterm infants. Since surfactant production only starts in the last three weeks or so of pregnancy, any baby born before 37 weeks is in danger from surfactant deficiency. Because surfactant stabilizes the inflated alveolus, a deficiency will cause failure of inflation and easy collapse of alveoli. The result is low compliance and poor ventilation with increased shunt.
  a) T The production of surfactant is normal at term (144.1).
  b) T A combination of factors contribute. The pulmonary vascular resistance is high in the fetus and also in the respiratorily distressed infant (144.1).
  c) T The severe hypoxia of respiratory distress causes a metabolic acidosis as well as a respiratory acidosis (144.1).
  d) T Note the phrase 'may be associated with'. If the infant undergoes positive pressure ventilation there will be a significant incidence of pneumomediastinum (144.1).
  e) T As in other intensive care situations, there is a balance to be struck between the oxygen needs of the body and the potential effects of oxygen toxicity (144.1).

145 Oxygen toxicity as a distinct entity is still subject to controversy.

Excessive inspired partial pressures of oxygen may cause:
a) retrolental fibroplasia
b) convulsions
c) Goodpasture's syndrome
d) proliferation of the type I alveolar cells
e) 'raptures of the deep'

146 Patients presenting for surgery may have concurrent cardiac disease which must be identified and treated to improve outcome. Hypertrophic cardiomyopathy seriously restricts cardiac output, especially in its end stages.

In hypertrophic (obstructive) cardiomyopathy:
a) there is usually an abnormal pressure gradient across the aortic valve
b) the left ventricular ejection fraction will be reduced
c) there may be autosomal recessive inheritance
d) syncope is not a common presentation
e) increasing the afterload will tend to increase the obstruction

References
145.1 Ped Clin N Am (1987)   p 1487
145.2 Nunn   p 491–495
145.3 Nunn   p 327–328
145.4 Davidson   p 570–571

146.1 Stoelting   p 151–155
146.2 Souhami & Moxham   p 418–419

145a) T Also known as retinopathy of prematurity, there is a contribution from high retinal artery oxygen tensions (145.1, 145.2).

b) T Partial pressures of oxygen above 2 atm (202 kPa) cause convulsions, which is the reason that divers use low FiO_2 at high ambient pressures (145.3).

c) F Goodpasture's syndrome is an autoimmune condition of the renal basement membrane with an element of cross-reactivity with the pulmonary alveolar membrane, resulting in poor oxygen transport (145.4).

d) F In pulmonary oxygen toxicity, the type I cells regress with a proliferation of the type II cells (145.2).

e) F 'Raptures of the deep' is a stage of nitrogen narcosis, not oxygen toxicity (145.3).

146 Hypertrophic obstructive cardiomyopathy (HOCM) tends to involve the septal wall and the mitral valve, producing syncope, angina, mitral regurgitation and exertional dyspnoea with high voltage ECG complexes.

a) F The gradient is subvalvular, the valve itself is normal (146.1).

b) F Left ventricular ejection fraction (LVEF) is often increased in HOCM and may reach 80% compared to a normal of about 60%. The ventricular volume may be markedly reduced, along with the stroke volume, but the fraction ejected is elevated (146.1, 146.2).

c) F There is an inherited element to HOCM, autosomal dominant rather than recessive (146.1).

d) F Syncope is one of the more common presentations (146.1).

e) F The obstruction tends to increase with reductions in afterload. Vasodilator drugs must be used with extreme care (146.1)

147 Chronic liver disease can result from many causes, including infections, drugs and alcohol. The end result is the same, a nodular, shrunken liver.

Clinical signs of chronic liver disease include:
a) central cyanosis
b) breast atrophy in women
c) gynaecomastia in men
d) testicular atrophy
e) enlargement of the parotid gland

148 Candidates must be familiar with the working principles of common monitoring equipment, including more recent developments, such as pulse oximetry. Recent journal reports have emphasized the fallibility of oximeters.

A pulse oximeter may give erroneous readings if:
a) there is significant methaemoglobinaemia
b) there is significant tricuspid incompetence
c) there is carboxyhaemoglobinaemia
d) there is a high concentration of HbF
e) the patient has dark coloured skin

References

147.1 Davidson   p 520–521

148.1 BJA (1992) 68   p 146–150
148.2 Miller   p 1138–1140
148.3 Miller   p 981–989

147a) T Central cyanosis is caused by increased intrapulmonary shunting due to high circulating bilirubin concentrations (147.1).
  b) T This completion and the next seem to be mutually exclusive, but they are both true. The reason is unclear but may involve sex-based imbalances in oestrogen and testosterone metabolism (147.1).
  c) T See b (147.1).
  d) T Testicular atrophy is part of the sex hormone imbalance. Oestrogen excess suppresses the function of the testis and causes atrophy (147.1).
  e) T (147.1).

148 Pulse oximetry has become an essential part of anaesthetic monitoring. Pulse oximeters measure the absorption of two wavelengths of light (920 and 660 nm) by the two main species of haemoglobin — oxyhaemoglobin and reduced haemoglobin. The other species of haemoglobin have their own absorption spectra which may influence the result. The absorbance of tissue is discounted by only displaying that for the pulsatile element, on the assumption that arterial pulsation is the only source for this.
  a) T Methaemoglobin has a high absorbance at 940 nm but an absorbance similar to oxyhaemoglobin at 660 nm. Above 85% saturation the reading is lower than expected, whereas below this level saturation is overestimated (148.2).
  b) T In tricuspid incompetence, the venous system is subjected to the pulsations of the right ventricle which causes retrograde pulsation in the capillary bed, confusing the instrument (148.3).
  c) T The absorption of carboxyhaemoglobin is similar to that of oxyhaemoglobin at 660 nm but low at 920 nm. The end result is an erroneously high reading (148.3).
  d) F There are few situations, apart from infancy where HbF is present in high concentrations. The absorbance of HbF is similar to HbA at the two measured wavelengths and so the reading of the monitor is unaffected (148.2).
  e) F Dark skin does not absorb light at the relevant frequencies and so makes no difference (148.3).

149 The oxygen–haemoglobin dissociation curve is met in all parts of the diploma examination. Candidates are advised to be able to draw the curve on demand and label it.

In the oxygen–haemoglobin dissociation curve, the P$_{50}$:
a) is the partial pressure of oxygen at which haemoglobin is 50% saturated
b) gives an indication of oxygen availability to the tissues
c) is decreased by acidosis
d) is increased if red cell 2, 3-diphosphoglycerate levels are low
e) if increased, is associated with an increase in the oxygen affinity of haemoglobin

150 Do not guess when confronted by daunting material. If necessary, read the references before attempting the question.

The following are consistent with a diagnosis of chronic haemolysis:
a) increased reticulocyte count
b) increased plasma conjugated bilirubin
c) increased urine bilirubin
d) increased faecal stercobilinogen
e) increased urine urobilinogen

References

149.1	Stoelting	p 558–560
149.2	Scurr, Feldman & Soni	p 491–493
150.1	Davidson	p 716–725
150.2	Davidson	p 502–503

149 The oxygen–haemoglobin dissociation curve is sigmoid. The position in relation to the x-axis (partial pressure of oxygen) determines the P_{50}, the partial pressure at which the haemoglobin is 50% saturated. The position of the curve, and therefore the P_{50}, is altered by phenomena that increase or decrease the affinity of haemoglobin for oxygen. If the affinity is increased then unloading of oxygen in the periphery is reduced, and vice-versa (149.1, 149.2).

a) **T** See above (149.1, 149.2).

b) **T** See above (149.1, 149.2)).

c) **F** The P_{50} is increased by acidosis, moving the curve to the right, reducing the affinity and increasing oxygen unloading in the periphery (149.1, 149.2)).

d) **F** Low levels of 2, 3-DPG shift the curve to the left, reducing the P_{50}, increasing oxygen affinity and reducing peripheral oxygen availability. This most commonly occurs after significant blood transfusion (149.1, 149.2).

e) **F** The opposite is true (149.1, 149.2).

150 Chronic (as opposed to acute) haemolysis leads to profound alterations in the metabolic pathways for both haemoglobin and bilirubin. Red cells destroyed by haemolysis are replaced in the long term by increased production of new red cells. The shortened maturation process results in immature cells (reticulocytes) being released into the general circulation. The haemoglobin released from the lysed red cells is metabolized to bilirubin and its variants.

a) **T** See above (150.1).

b) **F** Because the bilirubin conjugation mechanism in the liver tends to be overloaded, the levels of unconjugated bilirubin rise, but not levels of conjugated bilirubin (150.1).

c) **F** Unconjugated bilirubin is poorly water soluble and so does not appear in the urine (150.2).

d) **T** There is increased biliary excretion of bilirubin and hence stercobilinogen (150.2).

e) **T** Urobilinogen is excreted in the urine (150.1).

151 Although many of the inherited disorders of metabolism have no particular relevance to anaesthesia, glucose-6-phosphate dehydrogenase deficiency is an exception.

In glucose-6-phosphate dehydrogenase deficiency, haemolysis may be precipitated by:
a) thiopentone
b) halothane
c) aspirin
d) curare (d-tubocurarine)
e) fentanyl

152 It is recommended that candidates read the whole of the referenced chapter before attempting this question.

Intracellular concentrations of 2, 3-diphosphoglycerate (2, 3-DPG) are:
a) reduced with adaptation to altitude
b) increased in patients with stable diabetes
c) reduced in stored blood, causing a fall in the oxygen affinity of the haemoglobin
d) increased in hypophosphataemia
e) reduced with intracellular alkalosis

References

151.1 Stoelting   p 565–566

152.1 Scurr, Feldman & Soni   p 491–497

151 Glucose-6-phosphate dehydrogenase deficiency is the most common of the erythrocyte enzyme disorders. The condition affects some 8% of American black males. There is a chronic haemolytic anaemia of varying severity. Drugs which form peroxides upon interaction with haemoglobin tend to precipitate haemolysis. These peroxides are normally neutralized by a system dependent upon G6PD, but in the absence of G6PD there may be acute haemolytic jaundice after exibition of these drugs. The drugs implicated include paracetamol, a range of antibiotics, antimalarials, vitamin K and methylene blue. Infection may also precipitate haemolysis.
   a) F   (151.1).
   b) F   (151.1).
   c) F   (151.1).
   d) F   (151.1).
   e) F   (151.1).

152 The interplay of 2, 3-DPG and oxygen carriage is complex and beyond the scope of this text. Suffice to say that conditions which cause acidosis tend also to reduce 2, 3-DPG concentrations and therefore increase the oxygen affinity of the haemoglobin, preventing peripheral unloading of oxygen. Alkalotic conditions have the opposite effect.
   a) F   In adaptation to altitude there is a tendency to respiratory alkalosis until the renal excretion of bicarbonate can increase sufficiently to compensate, which it never does completely. Alkalosis increases the 2, 3-DPG concentration and reduces oxygen affinity, increasing peripheral unloading (152.1).
   b) T   Diabetic patients have increased concentrations of Hb1c, which has a high oxygen affinity. This is balanced by increased 2, 3 DPG concentrations which lower the affinity of HbA. The P_{50} does not change (152.1).
   c) F   Stored blood has a low concentration of 2, 3-DPG and therefore a high oxygen affinity, preventing peripheral unloading (152.1).
   d) F   2, 3-DPG concentrations are reduced in hypophosphataemia, a situation most commonly encountered in parenteral nutrition or subnutritional states (152.1).
   e) F   2, 3-DPG concentrations are increased in alkalosis, improving tissue delivery of oxygen (152.1).

153 The two following questions are based on radiological diagnosis. It is once more emphasized that radiological interpretation falls within the scope of the examination and requires revision, ideally aided by a radiologist.

A mediastinal mass on a plain chest X-ray:
a) may be a normal parathyroid gland
b) may be a primary choriocarcinoma
c) may be an enlarged azygos vein
d) may be due to primary tuberculosis even if there is no other sign of a 'primary complex'
e) may occur in Cushing's disease

154 On plain chest X-ray, an air bronchogram:
a) may be normal in children
b) may occur if there is a pneumothorax
c) may occur on an expiratory film
d) may occur following radiotherapy
e) may occur in sarcoidosis

References

153.1	Grainger & Allison	p 185–212
153.2	Grainger & Allison	p 142
154.1	Grainger & Allison	p 154–155
154.2	Grainger & Allison	p 149–161

153a) F Normal parathyroid glands may be intrathoracic but are too small to be seen on plain radiographs (153.1).
b) T Difficult to believe but true nevertheless; a primary germ cell tumour (seminoma, ovarian dysgerminoma or choriocarcinoma) may arise in the mediastinum. Germ cell tissue is not always confined to the gonads (153.1).
c) T The azygos and hemiazygos venous systems provide collateral drainage around the inferior vena cava (most commonly in pregnancy) and may be so enlarged because of IVC obstruction that they become visible on chest X-ray (153.2).
d) T The 'primary complex' in tuberculosis is the combination of peripheral calcification or scarring, usually in the upper lobe, with enlarged mediastinal lymph nodes (153.1).
e) T Patients with Cushing's disease, or those who are obese for other reasons, may have significant mediastinal fat deposits visible on chest X-ray (153.1).

154 Air bronchogram is one of the most common findings on a chest X-ray. It occurs because of the change in radiodensity between the air in the bronchus and the surrounding tissue. There are occasions when an air bronchogram is normal but many more when it is not (154.1, 154.2).
a) T The airways appear more prominent in children, even on X-ray (154.1).
b) T In the presence of a pneumothorax, the lung parenchyma may be more dense because of atelectasis which will increase the difference in density between the bronchus and the surrounding tissue (154.1).
c) T On expiration, the density of the surrounding tissue is increased (154.1).
d) T Radiotherapy causes tissue scarring, increasing its density (154.1).
e) T Sarcoidosis may cause interstitial fibrosis (154.1).

155 *Clostridium botulinum* is widely found in nature and is present in garden soil. There are several types of the bacterium which produce differing toxins.

Clostridium botulinum:
a) is usually sensitive to penicillin
b) toxin spares the autonomic nervous system
c) toxin has a post-synaptic effect
d) paralysis caused by the toxin is reversible by neostigmine
e) toxin may be used therapeutically

156 Cholelithiasis is a common surgical problem. Stones may be composed of cholesterol (usually Western countries) or pigment (mainly in the Far East).

Gall stones may be associated with:
a) haemolytic anaemia
b) oral contraception
c) bile duct tumours
d) sclerosing cholangitis
e) chronic pancreatitis

References
155.1 Souhami & Moxham   p 268
155.2 Souhami & Moxham   p 948
155.3 Prescribers Journal (1991) 31:5   p 197–201

156.1 Souhami & Moxham   p 641–642
156.2 Souhami & Moxham   p 615–619

155 *Clostridium botulinum* is an anaerobic bacterium producing a potent toxin which is usually found in inadequately cooked tinned meat or fish. Whilst rare in the UK, the incidence is considerably higher in some other countries because of differences in food preparation. The toxin binds permanently to presynaptic cholinergic nerve endings, and recovery is only possible because of the sprouting of new axonal fibres from the terminals. There are therapeutic uses for this toxin! (155.1, 155.2, 155.3).

a) **T** The organism itself is sensitive but it is the toxin which is the problem. The gut may have been colonized by the bacterium and so antibiotics may help in the prevention of further toxicity (155.2).

b) **F** The parasympathetic nervous system has cholinergic terminals which are also affected in botulism (155.1).

c) **F** See above. The toxin binds to the presynaptic membrane, preventing release of acetylcholine (155.2).

d) **F** If the presynaptic binding prevents the release of acetylcholine, then neostigmine can have no effect (155.2).

e) **T** Botulinum toxin has been used in the treatment of a variety of spastic muscle conditions, including squints and torticollis (155.3).

156a) T The haemolytic anaemias present a high bilirubin load to the gall bladder, altering the solubility of bilirubin and bile salts and causing pigment stones (156.1).

b) **T** The association exists and is probably due to altered hepatic metabolism (156.1).

c) **T** Whether this is because of otosis, trauma or alteration of the chemical environment is questionable (156.1).

d) **F** The cause of sclerosing cholangitis is not known. Multiple inflammatory stenoses are seen in the biliary tree. It does not seem to be associated with gall stones (156.1).

e) **T** Both acute and chronic pancreatitis are associated with gall stones, either as cause or effect (156.2).

157 The prevalence of infection with Human Immunodeficiency Virus (HIV) is rising. Wide knowledge of the condition is essential for the practising anaesthetist.

Infection with the Human Immunodeficiency Virus (HIV):
a) may present with a motor polyneuropathy
b) seborrhoeic dermatitis is a common feature
c) in cellular terms is confined to the T4 lymphocyte
d) may cause dementia
e) may cause ataxia

158 Peripheral nerve injury may follow:
a) shoulder dislocation
b) fracture of the tibia
c) fracture of the fibula
d) dislocation of the hip
e) fracture of the shaft of the humerus

References

157.1	Souhami & Moxham	p 965–966
157.2	Souhami & Moxham	p 250–254
157.3	Souhami & Moxham	p 1126
158.1	Gray	p 1136–1137
158.2	Gray	p 1148–1150

157 AIDS is an emotive subject. The majority of media coverage concerns primary prevention by behaviour modification. Clinical features of the disease get much less coverage, excepting the most common form of death which seems to be a major wasting illness with *Pneumocystis* pneumonia superimposed.
  a) **T** Motor polyneuropathy is common (157.1).
  b) **T** Seborrhoeic dermatitis is one of the many features of the aids related complex (ARC), a condition falling between asymptomatic infection and full AIDS but just as lethal (157.3).
  c) **F** Most information relates to T4 'helper' lymphocytes being colonized and later killed by HIV replication. Other immune cells are also involved, including monocytes and macrophages (157.2).
  d) **T** Cerebral effects, from aseptic meningitis and encephalitis to dementia are regular and often early features (157.1).
  e) **T** Ataxia is another of the encephalopathic features of HIV infection (157.1).

158a) T The axillary (circumflex humeral) nerve is at risk in fracture or dislocation of the shoulder; indeed, testing its function before reduction is a medico-legal necessity. Damage to this nerve causes a small patch of anaesthesia over the insertion of the deltoid muscle (158.1).
  b) **F** The nerves which pass through the lower limb are not usually in danger from fractures of the tibia (158.2).
  c) **T** The common peroneal (lateral popliteal) nerve is one of the most commonly injured nerves. It winds around the head of the fibula in an exposed position. The nerve may also be injured by lithotomy poles. Injury causes foot drop (158.2).
  d) **T** The sciatic nerve has a close posterior relation to the hip joint and may be injured by posterior dislocation or fracture-dislocation (158.2).
  e) **T** The radial nerve winds around the shaft of the humerus; it is palpable as it does so, and can be injured by fracture or pressure at this site (158.1).

159 The occurrence of headache after dural puncture (PDPH) is a major limitation on the use of spinal anaesthesia. Some recent developments in needle design are proving useful in reducing the incidence of PDPH.

The incidence of post dural puncture headache:
a) increases with age
b) is increased if a continuous catheter technique is used
c) is increased in females
d) is reduced if needles with solid tips are used
e) is reduced if the patient lies supine for 24 hours after dural puncture

160 Systemic arterial hypertension, both treated and untreated, is common in the surgical population. Interactions between the condition, the treatment and anaesthetic agents must be considered.

Persistent arterial hypertension may cause:
a) headache
b) left ventricular hypertrophy
c) dementia
d) retinal exudates
e) microscopic haematuria

References
159.1 Miller   p 1394
159.2 BJA (1991) 67:6   p 674–677

160.1 Souhami & Moxham   p 440–444
160.2 Souhami & Moxham   p 902
160.3 Souhami & Moxham   p 864–865
160.4 Souhami & Moxham   p 792–794
160.5 Davidson   p 316–322

159 The cause and incidence of post dural puncture headache (PDPH or spinal headache) varies from paper to paper. Most sources agree upon the cause — low cerebrospinal fluid pressure because of leakage through the puncture. Because of methodological differences, only generalizations can be drawn from papers comparing incidence when there are variations in technique. It can be said that the incidence is higher in the younger age groups, in women and in pregnancy, higher after labour than elective caesarean section, and higher with bigger needles and with needles which have a cutting tip with an end hole, compared to solid tips and side holes (159.1, 159.2).

a) F The contrary is true, the incidence falls with age, probably because the compliance of the intracranial contents falls (159.1, 159.2).

b) F (159.1).

c) T (159.1, 159.2).

d) T In theory, a Whitacre or Sprötte tip will separate the dural fibres rather than cutting them, and therefore the fibres can close back together afterward (159.1, 159.2).

e) F Lying supine will relieve the headache (because it is postural in nature). Lying supine will not shorten the time course of the headache in any way. Early mobilization will speed the onset of headache (159.1, 159.2).

160a) T It was once thought that headaches were a symptom of hypertension, but it is now realized that headache is no more common in the hypertensive patient than in the normal, except in those with hypertensive encephalopathy (160.1, 160.5).

b) T Left ventricular hypertrophy is one of the ECG or radiological signs of the condition (160.1, 160.5).

c) F Hypertension causes confusion, coma and convulsions, but not dementia (160.2, 160.5).

d) T Exudates are a classical fundoscopic sign of hypertension (160.3, 160.5).

e) F Proteinuria may be the result of hypertensive renal damage, but haematuria is not usually seen (160.1, 160.4, 160.5).

161 In a patient with severe burns:
a) suxamethonium should be avoided
b) there may be an increased requirement for non-depolarizing muscle relaxants
c) there may be an increased requirement for anaesthetic induction agents
d) resuscitation should be with salt poor solutions
e) there may be myoglobinuria

162 Know the physical properties of the anaesthetic vapours available, those of recent historical interest and also those about to be marketed.

The following are flammable in oxygen:
a) methoxyflurane
b) enflurane
c) isoflurane
d) sevoflurane
e) halothane

References

161.1	Miller	p 414–415
161.2	Miller	p 427
161.3	Miller	p 1997
161.4	Miller	p 232
161.5	Recent Advances 15	p 155–172
162.1	Dundee, Clarke & McCaughey	p 103–113

161a) T There have been a number of cardiac arrests because of the interactions between burned patients, suxamethonium and hyperkalaemia. This is said to be because of the increased density of receptors which develop on muscle membranes between one week and two months after injury (161.1).

b) T Posslbly due to the receptor change outlined above in **a** or because of the massive changes in fluid distribution (161.2, 161.3).

c) F The requirement for anaesthetic induction agents is lower than normal, as with any shocked patient (161.4).

d) F Burned patients lose sodium in large quantities from their wounds and require salt rich fluid as replacement (161.5).

e) T Myoglobin is released from damaged muscle. In deep burns, myoglobinuria may cause renal failure (161.5).

162 Nitrous oxide will support combustion <u>even in the absence of oxygen</u>.

a) T At a concentration of 5.4% in oxygen or 7% in air (162.1).

b) F Not in oxygen or air but at a concentration of 5.75% in nitrous oxide (162.1).

c) F (162.1).

d) T At a concentration of 11% in oxygen. Sevoflurane is not flammable in air (162.1).

e) F Not in oxygen or air but at 4.75% in nitrous oxide (162.1).

163 Etomidate is a commercially available induction agent in a solution with 35% propylene glycol at a concentration of 2 mg/ml.

Etomidate:
a) is soluble in water
b) potentiates non-depolarizing muscle relaxants
c) increases systemic vascular resistance
d) increases cerebral blood flow
e) inhibits plasma cholinesterase

164 The interactions of the anaesthetic vapours with soda lime are important clinical considerations.

The following undergo chemical reaction with soda lime under clinical conditions:
a) trichlorethylene
b) halothane
c) enflurane
d) isoflurane
e) sevoflurane

References

163.1 Dundee, Clarke & McCaughey   p 155–159

164.1 Dundee, Clarke & McCaughey   p 105–117

163 Etomidate is an imidazole derivative, notorious for pain on injection, involuntary movements and adrenal suppression. Etomidate has also become established as the usual agent in the precarious emergency case, because it seems to have a wider margin of safety than the barbiturates.

   a) T Etomidate is soluble in water, but the solution is too unstable for clinical use (163.1).

   b) T (163.1).

   c) F Systemic vascular resistance is reduced (163.1).

   d) F Intracranial pressure is reduced, hence the use of etomidate by infusion in severe head injury which has ceased since it became known that patients died from adrenal suppression (163.1).

   e) T Etomidate is both a competitive and noncompetitive inhibitor of plasma cholinesterase (163.1).

164 Read the question! The stem looks for chemical reaction, not clinically significant chemical reaction.

   a) T The products are phosgene, dichloroacetylene and hydrochloric acid (164.1).

   b) T 2-bromo-2-chloro-1, 1-difluoroethylene is the product. It is toxic but fortunately only produced in small, clinically insignificant quantities (164.1).

   c) F (164.1).

   d) F (164.1).

   e) T The products are not thought to be toxic. It seems a pity that such a promising new agent with potential for closed circuit use has this drawback (164.1).

165 In the fetal circulation:
a) the pulmonary vascular resistance falls at birth
b) the right atrial pressure is higher than the left
c) the extra-abdominal umbilical cord vessels have an autonomic nerve supply
d) all blood from the umbilical vein drains directly into the inferior vena cava
e) the foramen secundum is the orifice in the septum secundum

166 Thiopentone has been the most widely used induction agent since its introduction in 1934. Its popularity has been threatened by the introduction of the young pretender to the throne, 2, 6-diisopropyl phenol.

Thiopentone:
a) is highly protein bound
b) is highly ionized at plasma pH
c) is largely excreted unchanged in the urine
d) reduces the tone of the gravid uterus
e) may cause bronchospasm

References		
165.1 Miller		p 1876–1878
165.2 Gray		p 723–725
165.3 Gray		p 209–210
166.1 Dundee, Clarke & McCaughey		p 142–154

165a) T Before birth, the fetus is oxygenated by the placenta. The lungs are collapsed and have only a small blood supply. After birth the lungs expand and the high vascular resistance falls. This has further effects upon the distribution of blood between the aorta and pulmonary tree (165.1).

  b) T The difference in pressure between the atria is one of the reasons for the distribution of inferior vena caval blood to the left ventricle, and superior vena caval blood to the right ventricle (165.2).

  c) F The umbilical vessels have no nerve supply. The muscle in the vessels responds to physical changes, such as cold, pH, and handling, but not to neural influences (165.2).

  d) F Blood from the umbilical vein is distributed throughout the liver via the portal system, although some goes directly into the IVC via the ductus venosus (165.2).

  e) F Cardiac embryology is complex. The atria develop as one cavity. The septum primum develops centrally, separating the two atria. As this membrane reaches the atrioventricular cushion, the original orifice, the foramen primum, closes. To maintain flow between the two atria, a further foramen develops in the septum primum. This is the foramen secundum. Later, a further membrane, the septum secundum, develops to cover the foramen secundum without fusing to it. This provides the 'flap valve' effect which allows blood from the right atrium to flow into the left atrium under the influence of a pressure difference (165.3).

166a) T 60–85% of thiopentone is protein bound (166.1).

  b) F The vast majority of thiopentone is unionized at plasma pH (166.1).

  c) F Thiopentone undergoes extensive hepatic metabolism before being excreted in the urine. Only a very small proportion is excreted unchanged (166.1).

  d) F Thiopentone has no significant influence on the tone of the gravid uterus (166.1).

  e) T Bronchospasm is one of the features of anaphylactoid reaction to thiopentone (166.1).

167 Do not confuse closing capacity with closing volume; the two are not identical.

The closing capacity:
a) is the maximum lung volume at which airway closure can be detected in the dependent parts of the lung
b) is the same as the closing volume
c) cannot be measured unless the subject is awake and cooperative
d) may be measured using 100% oxygen as the tracer gas
e) is less than the functional residual capacity in a young adult

168 Water:
a) is highly ionized
b) has a pH of 7.0
c) has a dissociation constant of 1.8×10^{-16}
d) has a specific heat of 4186.8 J/kg
e) has a specific heat of 1 cal/g

References

167.1	Nunn	p 60–71
168.1	Harper	p 13–15
168.2	Dunnill & Colvin	p 236

167a) T (167.1).
  b) F The closing volume is the closing capacity minus the residual volume (167.1).
  c) F The closing capacity can be measured in anaesthetized, paralysed patients in much the same way as in awake individuals (167.1).
  d) T This is one of the 'tracer washout' methods of measurement. In principle, the subject inhales a single breath of tracer gas, starting at residual volume, and breathes out slowly through an analyser. At closing capacity the dependent airways close (having been closed at the beginning of the test they contain no tracer gas) and the concentration of trace gas rises because it is being washed out from the upper, open airways. If oxygen is used then it is nitrogen output which is measured (167.1).
  e) T With advancing age, the closing capacity begins to fall within the FRC, and airways start to close during quiet breathing (167.1).

168 Water is so universal that its properties are not often considered. In this question, water should be considered as pure (no additives or ions).
  a) F Water is ionized to a negligible extent. Ion generation may occur due to specific chemical reaction but in the normal state this is not the case (168.1). The probability of hydrogen existing as an ion in pure water is 0.0000000018.
  b) T There being equal concentrations of hydrogen ion and hydroxyl ion, as there must if a water molecule dissociates, the pH of water will be 7.0 (168.1).
  c) T (168.1).
  d) T (168.1, 168.2).
  e) T (168.1, 168.2).

169 A suitable electrocardiogram monitor will:
   a) have high- and low-pass filters in parallel
   b) have a band-pass filter set to accept frequencies of 0.1 to 50 Hz
   c) have common mode rejection
   d) have a mains isolation transformer
   e) share a common earth with other electrical equipment

170 Inotropic agents are employed frequently in intensive care units. Apart from the time honoured agents (such as dopamine), knowledge of the newer drugs, enoximone for example, will prove useful.

When considering positive inotropic drugs:
   a) the optical isomers of dobutamine have different properties
   b) dobutamine tends to cause venodilatation
   c) dopamine has a greater chronotropic effect than dobutamine
   d) dopamine increases myocardial oxygen demand
   e) isoprenaline has a significant alpha adrenergic action

References

169.1	Miller	p 968–974
169.2	Scurr, Feldman & Soni	p 52–65
170.1	Goodman & Gilman	p 200–203
170.2	Dundee, Clarke & McCaughey	p 351–360

169 An ECG monitor, as opposed to a <u>diagnostic</u> machine, has two roles: first, to amplify and display the small electrical voltage changes of the ECG sequence without interference; and second, to prevent accidental electric shock. To achieve the first requires an amplifier which has a filter mechanism to reject unwanted frequencies without loss of signal quality. To achieve the second requires Isolation from mains voltages and induced currents.

a) F If two filters are included in the machine, one set to reject high frequencies and the other set to reject low frequencies, with the two in series then the effect will be that of a 'band-pass' filter. This will restrict the unwanted noise and reduce the interference with the signal. Setting the two in parallel will have no effect (169.1, 169.2).

b) T (169.1, 169.2).

c) T Common mode rejection is a system whereby only the <u>difference</u> in voltage between two leads will be measured, rather than the <u>actual</u> voltage. This system rejects any voltage common to both leads, cleaning the signal somewhat (169.1, 169.2).

d) T The theory is that any equipment in contact with the patient is isolated from the mains to prevent electric shock (169.1, 169.2).

e) T If there were differences in the earths between different equipment, there could be different voltages on each earth lead, with the possibility of electric shock (169.1, 169.2).

170a) T (+)– dobutamine is a potent alpha antagonist whereas (–)– dobutamine is an alpha agonist. The (+)– isomer is a more potent beta agonist than is the (–)– isomer (170.1).

b) T (170.2).

c) T (170.2).

d) T Both dopamine and dobutamine increase myocardial oxygen supply, but dopamine also increases oxygen demand (170.2).

e) F Isoprenaline has almost no alpha activity (170.2).

171 The factors affecting cerebral blood flow should be familiar. Take care when considering the specific wording of some completions.

Cerebral blood flow (CBF):
a) is increased by raised Pa_{CO_2}
b) is increased by raising pH in the extracellular fluid
c) during persistent hyperventilation, CBF increases after an initial fall
d) is decreased by raising Pa_{O_2}
e) the effect of low Pa_{CO_2} in reducing CBF over-rides the effect of low Pa_{O_2} in increasing CBF

172 The absolute contraindications to lumbar epidural anaesthesia include:
a) chronic neurological disease
b) previous laminectomy at the L5 level
c) bleeding diathesis with INR greater than 2.0
d) a history of poliomyelitis
e) abruptio placenta

References

171.1	Scurr, Feldman & Soni	p 208–209
172.1	Stoelting	p 314–315
172.2	Miller	p 847
172.3	Miller	p 1378
172.4	Macintosh	p 183–184
172.5	Wildsmith	p 38–40
172.6	Synopsis	p 691–692

171a) T (171.1).

b) F The cerebral blood flow (CBF) is increased by a <u>fall</u> in pH (171.1).

c) T Hyperventilation, with reduction of Pa_{CO_2}, is often used as a means of reducing CBF and intracranial pressure. This effect is short-lived and the CBF returns to its previous level after a short, variable period (171.1)

d) F Increasing the Pa_{O_2} from normal does not effect the CBF. Reducing the Pa_{O_2} from normal increases the CBF (171.1).

e) F The effect of low Pa_{O_2} overrides the effect of low Pa_{CO_2} (171.1).

172a) F Chronic neurological disease is a relative contraindication in that most chronic neurological diseases follow a relapsing and remitting course, usually relapsing at times of stress such as surgery or childbirth. If a regional anaesthetic technique is used, the patient may blame the anaesthetist for the relapse when they are only coincident (post hoc sed non propter hoc – after it but not because of it) (172.1, 172.2,172.5).

b) F Previous surgery or scoliosis merely mean that the technique may be difficult or the anaesthesia not adequate because of altered distribution. There is no absolute contraindication (172.5, 172.6).

c) T One of the few absolute contraindications. There is always a risk of perforation of an epidural vessel, and in the presence of a bleeding tendency an epidural haematoma may form causing cord compression. Some debate exists about patients whose INR lies between 1 and 1.5 and those receiving aspirin or subcutaneous heparin. There is no debate about INR values greater than 2. Reference (172.4) suggests this as a relative rather than absolute contraindication (172.1, 172.2, 172.3, 172.4, 172.5).

d) F Poliomyelitis causes destruction of anterior horn cells in the acute phase of the disease. It is not necessary to avoid epidural anaesthesia in later life (172.2, 172.5).

e) T Epidural anaesthesia in the presence of unresuscitated hypovolaemia is contraindicated because of the precipitate hypotension which may ensue (172.6).

173 Knowledge of the Glasgow Coma Scale is essential for the accurate assessment of head injury.

In the assessment of head injury:
a) a higher Glasgow Coma Score indicates more serious coma
b) extensor movements in response to pain are more serious than flexor movements
c) spontaneous hyperventilation is a sign of increased intracranial pressure
d) assessment of verbal responses is a part of the Glagow Coma Scale
e) arterial hypotension may indicate rising intracranial pressure

174 Familial multiple polyposis coli (Gardener's syndrome):
a) may be associated with osteoma
b) may undergo malignant change
c) may be associated with epidermoid cysts
d) is inherited as a recessive condition
e) does not develop adenomatous lesions outside the colon

References

173.1	Miller	p 1987
173.2	Miller	p 1756
173.3	Nimmo & Smith	p 1438–1441
174.1	Souhami & Moxham	p 596–597
174.2	Davidson	p 471–472

173a) F The reverse is true. Higher scores indicate better function, lower scores indicate poorer function (173.1, 173.2).
b) T With deteriorating condition of the patient, flexor movements give way to spontaneous extensor movements (173.1, 173.2).
c) T The presence of spontaneous hyperventilation can be used as an indication for mechanical ventilation of the lungs (173.3).
d) T (173.1, 173.2).
e) F Increasing intracranial pressure tends to cause arterial hypertension rather than hypotension (173.3).

174 Familial polyposis coli is an inherited tendency to develop large numbers of colonic adenomata. The adenomata appear after puberty and may undergo malignant change within 15 years. Prophylactic panprocto-colectomy is one means of management. There are a number of recognized associations of the condition.
a) T The association is part of Gardener's syndrome (174.1, 174.2).
b) T Malignant change is the most widely known feature of the condition (174.1, 174.2).
c) T (174.1, 174.2).
d) F Autosomal dominant inheritance (174.1, 174.2).
e) F Development of stomach and small intestinal polyps which may also become malignant is well known (174.1, 174.2).

175 A huge array of drugs may cause embarrassment to the bone marrow.
The following may be associated with agranulocytosis·
a) cimetidine
b) trimethoprim
c) diclofenac
d) cephalosporins
e) etomidate

176 Pseudomembranous colitis is a condition of profuse watery diarrhoea due to the presence of the bacterium *Clostridium difficile*.
The following can cause pseudomembranous colitis:
a) gentamicin
b) vancomycin
c) imipenem
d) metronidazole
e) clindamycin

References

175.1	Goodman & Gilman	p 899–902
175.2	BNF	section 1.3.1
175.3	Data Sheet Compendium	p 1470
175.4	Goodman & Gilman	p 1052–1057
175.5	BNF	section 5.1.8
175.6	Data Sheet Compendium	p 930
175.7	Goodman & Gilman	p 669
175.8	Goodman & Gilman	p 1090
175.9	BNF	section 15.1.1
176.1	BNF	section 5.1.4
176.2	Goodman & Gilman	p 1135–1137
176.3	BNF	section 5.1.2

175a) T Cimetidine is very rarely associated with agranulocytosis, but the association is recognized to exist (175.1, 175.2, 175.3).
b) T Trimethoprim is well known for bone marrow suppression (175.4, 175.5).
c) T The association is referred to in the data sheet but not in ref (175 7) (175.6, 175.7).
d) T (175.8).
e) F Etomidate is infamous for adrenal suppression, but not bone marrow suppression (177.9)

176 Pseudomembranous colitis (PC) is a rare but severe condition following antibiotic therapy. There occurs overgrowth of colonic *Clostridium difficile*, which produces a mucosal toxin leading to diarrhoea.
a) T Most of the aminoglycoside antibiotics are known to cause this condition, excepting vancomycin (see below) (176.1).
b) F Vancomycin is the <u>treatment</u> for PC (176.2).
c) T Imipenem is a beta-lactam antibiotic usually prepared with cilastatin to reduce renal excretion of the active drug. It has been known to cause PC (176.3).
d) F Metronidazole can be used to treat PC (176.2).
e) T Clindamicin is the antibiotic most notorious for causing PC and was the first drug recognized as a cause for the condition (176.2).

177 In the spinal cord:
a) the dorsal columns convey vibration sense
b) temperature sense is carried in the spinothalamic tracts
c) proprioception is carried in the spinothalamic tracts
d) all touch sense is carried in the dorsal columns
e) the corticospinal tracts are a major motor pathway

178 Surgical diagnosis should not rely upon a single test. There are usually multiple causes for any single biochemical test result to be abnormal.

Elevated plasma amylase activity might be found in:
a) diabetic ketoacidosis
b) ruptured ectopic pregnancy
c) perforated peptic ulcer
d) severe glomerular impairment
e) intestinal obstruction

References

177.1 Souhami & Moxham   p 925

178.1 Zilva & Pannall   p 313–315

177a) **T** The dorsal columns transmit vibration sense (177.1).
  b) **T** The spinothalamic tract conveys temperature sensation (177.1).
  c) **F** Proprioception is a modality transmitted in the dorsal columns (177.1).
  d) **F** Touch is shared between the dorsal columns and the spinothalamic tract (177.1).
  e) **T** (177.1).

178 Amylase is usually thought of as a pancreatic enzyme. There are other significant sites of production, such as salivary gland, Fallopian tube, skeletal muscle, fat and gonads! Being of low molecular weight, the protein is excreted in urine; thus any cause of renal impairment may elevate the plasma activity. Any cause of acute abdominal pain may also have this effect. All these completions are true.
  a) **T** (178.1).
  b) **T** (178.1).
  c) **T** (178.1).
  d) **T** (178.1).
  e) **T** (178.1).

179 The associations of disease states may be numerous. Be especially wary of stating that a particular association does <u>not</u> exist.

Ankylosing spondylitis is associated with:
a) pulmonary fibrosis
b) conjunctivitis
c) aortic valve regurgitation
d) cardiac conduction abnormalities
e) uveitis

180 Inguinal field block is one of the most frequently performed local anaesthetic techniques. Applied anatomy is essential to the practice of safe and effective regional anaesthesia.

Inguinal field block may cause:
a) anaesthesia over the anterolateral part of the thigh
b) anaesthesia over the anteromedial part of the thigh
c) anaesthesia of the root of the penis
d) sufficient anaesthesia for circumcision
e) anaesthesia of the peritoneum sufficient for a hernia repair

References

179.1 Stoelting   p 636–637

180.1 Eriksson   p 107–108
180.2 Eriksson   p 52–54
180.3 Wildsmith   p 132–135

179 Although ankylosing spondylitis is generally viewed as a skeletal problem, with spinal rigidity as the main anaesthetic problem, there are a number of systemic effects. All these completions are true.
a) **T** (179.1).
b) **T** (179.1).
c) **T** (179.1).
d) **T** (179.1).
e) **T** (179.1).

180 Inguinal field block is one of the easiest regional techniques to perform. The area infiltrated contains the ilioinguinal and iliohypogastric nerves as they pass superior and then medial to the iliac spine before supplying the lower anterior abdominal wall and the inguinal canal, spermatic cord and testicle.
a) **T** the anterolateral surface of the thigh is supplied by the lateral cutaneous nerve of the thigh, which passes under (or through) the inguinal ligament near the iliac spine and so is likely to become involved in an inguinal field block where this area is infiltrated (180.1).
b) **F** The femoral branch of the genitofemoral nerve supplies the anteromedial aspect of the thigh. The nerve does not become involved in this particular technique (180.2).
c) **T** The iliohypogastric nerve supplies the lower abdominal wall, including the root of the penis (180.3), and will be blocked in the inguinal field technique.
d) **F** The skin of most of the penis is supplied by the dorsal penile nerves, branches of the pudendal nerves. These are not involved in the technique described (180.3).
e) **F** The peritoneum must be infiltrated separately (180.2).

181 Flumazenil:
   a) is a benzodiazepine
   b) has extensive protein binding
   c) has a plasma elimination half-life of less than one hour
   d) accelerates recovery from halothane anaesthesia
   e) will antagonize the effects of phenytoin

182 Haematuria may be defined loosely as the presence of blood in the urine. Remember that it may be macro- or microscopic.

Haematuria may occur in the following:
   a) subacute bacterial endocarditis
   b) sickle cell disease
   c) polycystic kidney
   d) acute intermittent porphyria
   e) blackwater fever

References

181.1 Dundee, Clarke & McCaughey   p 190–191

182.1 Davidson   p 556
182.2 Souhami & Moxham   p 825
182.3 Davidson   p 153–154
182.4 Souhami & Moxham   p 781–782
182.5 Souhami & Moxham   p 299

181 Flumazenil is a specific benzodiazepine receptor antagonist which does not alter plasma drug concentrations. It also antagonizes the effects of alcohol (athough the manufacturers do not emphasize the point).
- **a) T** Flumazenil is an imidazobenzodiazepine (181.1).
- **b) F** Only about 40% of flumazenil is protein bound (181.1).
- **c) T** (181.1)
- **d) T** Although the mechanism is not yet clear (181.1)
- **e) F** Flumazenil is an antagonist to benzodiazepines. The action of phenytoin is not antagonized (181.1).

182 The investigation of haematuria demands a detailed knowledge of the structure and function of the whole urinary tract. Haematuria is the presence of blood, i.e. intact red cells, in the urine. Haemoglobinuria implies free haemoglobin rather than red cells and has different causes.
- **a) T** (182.1).
- **b) T** (182.1).
- **c) T** Haematuria is one of the more common presentations of polycystic kidney (182.1, 182.2).
- **d) F** In acute intermittent porphyria, the urine becomes dark on standing because of the presence of excess porphobilinogen in urine, not true haematuria (182.1, 182.4).
- **e) F** Black water fever is a haemolytic complication of malaria, where the haemolysis is so severe that the urine becomes dark from haemoglobinuria. There is no haematuria as such (182.3, 182.5).

183 There remains a degree of residual uncertainty over the breakdown pathway of atracurium.

The metabolism of atracurium:
a) is predominantly by Hofmann elimination
b) is inhibited in hypothermia
c) is inhibited by increasing blood pH
d) produces a metabolite with muscle relaxant activity
e) produces a metabolite with vagolytic activity

184 Chronic lead poisoning is less frequently met since the change of plumbing material from lead to copper. Patients with the protean features of poisoning with heavy metals may, however, still present.

Chronic lead poisoning may cause:
a) gastroenteritis
b) a blue line on the gums
c) emphysema
d) peripheral neuropathy
e) renal failure

References

183.1 Dundee, Clarke & McCaughey   p 307–308

184.1 Souhami & Moxham   p 67
184.2 Davidson   p 91

183a) F Although the molecule does undergo Hofmann elimination (a spontaneous breakdown under specific conditions of temperature and pH) the predominant metabolic pathway is by ester hydrolysis (183.1).

  b) T Falling temperature reduces the breakdown of the molecule, hence the recommendation of refrigerated storage (183.1).

  c) F Metabolism and breakdown are reduced by falling pH, hence the storage in a medium adjusted to pH 3.5 (183.1).

  d) T Metabolism of atracurium results in two main metabolites, laudanosine and a quaternary monoacrylate. The monoacrylate has neuromuscular blocking activity (183.1) .

  e) T The monoacrylate metabolite has vagolytic activity as well as muscle relaxant activity (183.1). See above.

184a) T All the heavy metals cause gastrointestinal symptoms, usually diarrhoea and colicky abdominal pain (184.1, 184.2).

  b) T A gum line does occur with lead but is much more common with other metals such as mercury (184.1, 184.2).

  c) F Emphysema and asthma tend to occur with cadmium, chromium, vanadium and platinum poisoning rather than lead (184.1).

  d) T The neuropathy is usually motor. Polyneuropathy also occurs with thallium, bismuth and arsenic poisoning (184.1, 184.2).

  e) T Renal impairment also occurs with thallium, bismuth and arsenic poisoning (184.1).

185 The Vaughan-Williams classification of anti-arrhythmic agents is commonly met in examination papers. A revision table on this subject will repay the effort.

Class I anti-arrhythmic drugs:
a) may prolong the intracellular action potential
b) may shorten the intracellular action potential
c) may have no effect upon the intracellular action potential
d) include the beta blockers
e) potentiate fast sodium current

186 Second degree heart block:
a) is usually the result of disease above the atrio-ventricular node
b) in Mobitz type II block there is a progressive increase in the P–R interval
c) in Mobitz type II block the P–R interval of the conducted beats is extended but constant
d) may be precipitated by verapamil
e) usually requires a permanent pacemaker

References

185.1 Davidson   p 273–276
185.2 Souhami & Moxham   p 363–373

186.1 Davidson   p 273–279
186.2 Souhami & Moxham   p 360–363

185 The stem refers to the classification of anti-arrhythmic drugs by Singh and Vaughan-Williams (185.1, 185.2), which does not refer to anatomical site of action but to effect on action potentials. Class I drugs inhibit fast sodium channels in addition to their other actions. The first three of these completions may seem to be mutually exclusive. They are not; it depends which drug is used as the example.

    a) T The class Ia drugs — quinidine, procainamide and disopyramide — prolong the intracellular action potential (185.1, 185.2).

    b) T The class Ib drugs — lignocaine, mexelitine and phenytoin — shorten the action potential (185.1, 185.2).

    c) T The class Ic drug, flecanide has no effect upon the duration of the action potential (185.1, 185.2).G

    d) F The beta blockers are not class I drugs but class II (185.1, 185.2).

    e) F The class I antiarrhythmics inhibit fast sodium channels rather than potentiating them (185.1, 185.2).

186 There are two types of second degree heart block, Mobitz types I and II. Type I is the Wenckebach phenomenon, where the P–R interval increases progressively beat to beat until a beat is dropped. In type II block the P–R interval of the conducted beats is constant but occasional beats are dropped, usually in a regular manner.

    a) F Second degree heart block is due to disease in the conducting system, usually the A–V node itself (186.1, 186.2).

    b) F It is Mobitz type I block (the Wenckebach phenomenon) where the P–R interval increases until a beat is dropped (186.1, 186.2).

    c) F In Mobitz type II block the P–R interval of conducted beats is constant and normal, the dropped beat being unannounced (186.1, 186.2).

    d) T Verapamil is the first line treatment for supraventricular tachyarrhythmias and can precipitate or reveal second degree heart block if used generously (186.2).

    e) F Most patients with second degree heart block are unaware of it. There is not usually progression to complete heart block, which would require a pacemaker (186.1, 186.2).

187 Polycystic disease of the kidneys is a major maldevelopment of the renal tubules resulting in multiple cyst formation.

Adult polycystic disease of the kidney may be associated with:
a) arterial hypertension
b) cysts in the liver
c) renal failure
d) autosomal recessive inheritance
e) unilateral disease

188 The diaphragm:
a) receives all sensory supply from the phrenic nerves
b) has cross innervation by the two phrenic nerves
c) will become paralysed by a spinal cord transection at the C5 level
d) diaphragmatic pain may be referred to the dermatome of T1
e) the phrenic nerves spread across the pericardial surface before entering the muscle

---

References

187.1 Bullock, Sibley & Whitaker   p 64–65

188.1 Gray   p 592–595
188.2 Gray   p 1151
188.3 Davidson   p 437

107 Adult polycystic disease of the kidney is an autosomal dominant inherited disease of both kidneys presenting in the third or fourth decades. It may present with hypertension, renal masses or renal impairment. There is an association with hepatic cysts but without change in liver function. The adult condition must be distinguished from infantile polycystic kidney disease which features recessive inheritance and a high early mortality from renal, hepatic or respiratory failure, the latter because of mechanical restriction by the expanding cysts (187.1).

a) T See above (187.1).
b) T See above (187.1).
c) T See above (187.1).
d) F See above (187.1).
e) F See above (187.1).

188a) F While the phrenic nerves provide the majority of the sensory and motor supply to the diaphragm, there is a contribution from the intercostal nerves peripherally (188.1).
b) F Each phrenic nerve supplies its own half of the diaphragm with no cross innervation (188.1).
c) F The phrenic nerves arise from the cervical spinal cord at C3, C4, C5. A transection at C5 will spare the majority of the nerve (188.1).
d) F Diaphragmatic pain is said to be referred to the shoulder tip. The affected dermatome is either C4 or C5. Referred pain implies that the irritated organ and the affected dermatome have the same neural origin. The phrenic nerve has no contribution from T1 (188.2, 188.3).
e) F The phrenic nerves pierce the diaphragm before spreading across the peritoneal surface. The fibres then enter the muscle from below (188.1).

189 Circle absorber anaesthesia systems are gaining in popularity due to the increased use of the more expensive anaesthetic vapours, and environmental concerns. The properties of the absorbent are essential knowledge. Refer to question 164.

With regard to soda lime:
a) it will absorb a significant amount of halothane when dry
b) it contains 80% calcium hydroxide and 20% barium hydroxide
c) the reaction of carbon dioxide with soda lime produces calcium carbonate
d) the maximum absorption of carbon dioxide is 5 L/100g of absorbent
e) the colour change with use is the result of temperature change

190 The definition of minimal alveolar concentration (MAC) has been detailed earlier. Several factors elevate and reduce MAC.

The minimum alveolar concentration of halothane is reduced by:
a) ephedrine
b) iproniazid
c) clonidine
d) reserpine
e) methyldopa

References		
189.1 Miller	p 99	
189.2 Miller	p 195–196	
190.1 Aitkenhead & Smith	p 154	
190.2 BJA (1992) 68	p 123–125	
190.3 Dundee, Clarke & McCaughey	p 421–422	

189a) T Excessive absorption of halothane by dry soda lime can cause problems of prolonged induction, extended time to steady state and leaching of halothane during subsequent cases. This does not happen when the agent has been dampened by exhaled water (189.1).

b) F This is baralyme not soda lime. Soda lime contains 94% calcium hydroxide and 5% sodium hydroxide (189.2).

c) T After a complex reaction involving carbon dioxide, water, heat, sodium hydroxide and calcium hydroxide, one end product is calcium carbonate (189.2).

d) F The maximum is 26 litres but this is usually reduced to between 10 and 20 litres by channelling within the absorber (189.2).

e) F Whichever dye is used, the colour changes are pH dependent (189.2).

190 It is said that the centrally acting alpha 2 agonists — clonidine, reserpine and methyldopa — which decrease central adrenergic stores, all have the effect of reducing vapour requirements. References are few, 190.1 suggests that the opposite effect, an increase in requirement, is shown by ephedrine and the MAOI, iproniazid. Logic suggests that this should be so but confirmation is difficult to obtain.

a) F (190.1).

b) F (190.1).

c) T (190.2, 190.3).

d) T (190.2, 190.3).

e) T (190.2, 190.3).

191 The constituents of papaveretum relate to its biological origins. Recently there has been speculation over the possible teratogenic potential of noscapine.

Papaveretum contains:
a) morphine
b) dihydrocodeine
c) codeine
d) papaverine
e) diacetylmorphine

192 Opacity of the lens is more widely referred to as cataract.

Opacity of the lens may be associated with:
a) anorexia nervosa
b) diabetes
c) gonorrhoea
d) radiation
e) trachoma

References

191.1 Data Sheet Compendium   p 1272

192.1 OTM   p 23.18–19
192.2 Davidson   p 686
192.3 OTM   p 9.83–84
192.4 Souhami & Moxham   p 258–265

191 In late 1991, the Committee on Safety of Medicines circulated advice that papaveretum should not be given to females of childbearing potential. Evidence had accumulated that one of the components of the mixture, noscapine, caused polyploidy in mammalian cell culture lines. Papaveretum was then reformulated without the noscapine and rc launched in early 1992. The ingredients are now morphine, codeine and papaverine.
   a) **T** See above (191.1).
   b) **F** Codeine is present, not dihydrocodeine (191.1).
   c) **T** See above (191.1).
   d) **T** Papaverine is a smooth muscle antispasmodic, but not an analgesic. See above (191.1).
   e) **F** Diacetylmorphine is also known as diamorphine or heroin. It is a synthetic derivative of morphine. It is not present in papaveretum (191.1).

192a) T Lens opacification seems to be a part of the major metabolic upset which occurs in anorexia nervosa (192.1).
   b) **T** There is a rare form of cataract in young, unstable diabetic patients. The senile form is no more common in diabetic patients than in the non-diabetic population, except that it may appear earlier (192.2, 192.3).
   c) **F** Congenital gonorrhoea causes ophthalmia neonatorum, a purulent infection of the conjunctiva in which the lens is not involved (192.4).
   d) **T** There is little material in medical texts but the association seems to be with ultraviolet radiation rather than radioactivity (192.1). This is substantiated by the effects of UV radiation in Chile (caused by ozone depletion) which is causing widespread cataracts in sheep.
   e) **F** Trachoma is a chronic infection with *Chlamydia trachomatis* and causes conjunctivitis, fibrosis and scarring of the eyelids and eventually blindness because of corneal scarring (192.4).

193 Myasthenia gravis is an autoimmune disease characterized by exercise-induced fatigue of skeletal muscle.

In myasthenia gravis:
a) there may be asymmetric muscle weakness
b) thymic hyperplasia is rare
c) there is sensitivity to the aminoglycoside antibiotics
d) there are usually antibodies to acetylcholine
e) ptosis is a late sign

194 Microshock is dangerous for both patients and staff. The increasing use of electrical equipment in operating environments increases the risk.

To reduce the possibility of microshock to a patient:
a) electrical equipment connected to the patient must have an earth leakage current of more than 10 μA
b) any electrical circuits in contact with the patient should be isolated from earth
c) pacemaker leads should be handled with gloves
d) central venous catheters should be filled with saline solutions
e) electrical equipment should have a non-conductive coating

References

193.1	Stoelting	p 626–630
193.2	Souhami & Moxham	p 947–948
194.1	Sykes, Vickers & Hull	p 146–147

193 Myasthenia gravis affects the process of anaesthesia because of the unpredictability of patient response to muscle relaxants and respiratory depressant drugs, and because patients may come to surgery either for the condition itself or incidentally.

a) **T** Despite the disease being a systemic condition, there may be asymmetry in its effects, either left and right being unequally affected or shoulder girdle more than pelvis (193.1, 193.2).

b) **F** Some 70% of patients with myasthenia gravis have thymic hyperplasia. This may not show as thymic enlargement (193.1, 193.2).

c) **T** The aminoglycosides have muscle relaxant properties, and myasthenics are exquisitely sensitive to this (193.1).

d) **F** The antibodies in myasthenia gravis are to the cholinergic receptor site, not to acetylcholine itself (193.1).

e) **F** Ptosis is frequently a presenting feature of myasthenia gravis (193.1, 193.2).

194 Microshock is a situation where small electrical currents can be applied to the myocardium by accident, causing arrhythmia or death.

a) **F** The earth leakage current is the current measured between the live and the earth of a piece of equipment in normal use. If it is too high, then electric shock is possible if an alternate low resistance route to earth exists. 10 μA is the <u>maximum</u> acceptable current, not the minimum (194.1).

b) **T** If the patient circuit is isolated from earth then there is less opportunity for current to leak through the patient. The equipment itself should be earthed (194.1).

c) **T** Wearing gloves to handle pacemaker leads will prevent electrical contacts between the free end of the lead and the machine when the handler is in contact with both (194.1).

d) **F** Saline filled central venous catheters can act as good conductors of stray currents. They should be filled with a nonconductive fluid such as dextrose (194.1).

e) **T** If the equipment is coated with a nonconductive material, then there will be less oportunity for conduction by hand-to-hand contact (194.1).

195 Enoximone:
  a) decreases intramyocardial cyclicAMP concontrations
  b) maintenance dose is 20–40 µg/kg per min
  c) inhibits phosphodiesterase
  d) causes a rise in systemic vascular resistance
  e) is a bipyridine derivative

196 Watery bile is produced by the liver and later concentrated by water absorption. The addition of mucin by the gall bladder causes thickening.

Bile contains:
  a) amylase
  b) the potassium salts of bile acids
  c) unconjugated bilirubin
  d) cholesterol
  e) phospholipids

References

195.1 Dundee, Clarke & McCaughey   p 358–359

196.1 Zilva & Pannall   p 300–301

195 The 'standard' inotropes, dopamine and dobutamine, increase myocardial contractility by increasing intracellular cyclicAMP concentrations. This is achieved by stimulation of adrenergic receptors. Enoximone increases cyclicAMP concentrations by inhibiting its breakdown by phosphodiesterase (195.1).
   a) F Enoximone increases intracellular cyclicAMP concentrations. See above (195.1).
   b) F The maintenance dose is 5–20 μg/kg per min (195.1)
   c) T See above (195.1).
   d) F Enoximone causes a fall in systemic vascular resistance. See also question 107 (195.1).
   e) F Enoximone is an imidazolone derivative. Amrinone is an inotrope derived from bipyridine (195.1).

196 The function of bile is to act as an emulsifier for fat and fat-soluble nutrients in the small bowel. One to two litres of bile are produced by the liver daily. This is concentrated about 10 times in the gall bladder before passage to the gut. The bile acids which perform the emulsification undergo enterohepatic recirculation, so that the bile contains both primary and secondary bile salts (196.1).
   a) F Bile contains no enzymes (196.1).
   b) F Hepatic bile contains electrolytes at approximately plasma concentrations. After concentration in the gall bladder, the major cation is still sodium (196.1).
   c) F Unconjugated bilirubin is poorly water soluble and is conjugated in the liver to increase the solubility. Bile contains conjugated bilirubin (196.1).
   d) T Cholesterol is responsible for the commonest stones (196.1).
   e) T Phospholipids are present in bile (196.1).

197 The 'Guide to Training' issued by the Royal College of Anaesthetists suggests that some knowledge of the history of anaesthesia would be useful, though not essential. Refer to question 63

Historically:
a) Bier was the first to give a deliberate spinal anaesthetic
b) lignocaine was introduced in 1935
c) Wood described the hollow needle before the first description of inhalational anaesthesia
d) the first described use of cocaine as a local anaesthetic was by Freud
e) Bier described a single tourniquet method of intravascular local anaesthesia

198 The differences between the physical and chemical properties of various gases and vapours may be used to measure their concentrations.

The following properties may be used to measure the concentration of a gas or vapour:
a) the refractive index
b) the thermal conductivity
c) the solubility
d) light emission
e) light absorption

References

197.1	Macintosh	p 4–8
197.2	Atkinson, Rushman & Lee	p 35
197.3	Atkinson, Rushman & Lee	p 2–3
197.4	Arch Klin Chirugerie (1908) 86	p 1007
198.1	Sykes, Vickers & Hull	p 229–242

197 Local anaesthesia has as interesting a history as general anaesthesia, some 50 years later.

a) F Bier was the first to develop a reproducible method of spinal anaesthesia but he was not the first to achieve it. That honour fell to Corning, whose method is more likely to result in an epidural or paravertebral block. Corning used spinal injection of cocaine not to produce anaesthesia but as a method of relieving pain in such conditions as decompression sickness. (197.1).

b) F In 1947 (197.2).

c) F The hollow needle was described by Wood in 1853, some 10 years after inhalational anaesthesia became available (197.1).

d) F Freud suggested it, Koller did it, by instillation into the conjunctiva (197.3).

e) F Bier's original technique was to inject local anaesthetic into a vein in a section of limb isolated by tourniquets above and below the operation site (197.4).

198a) T The Rayleigh refractometer uses the differences in refractive index between vapours to assess concentration. The instrument compares the refraction of a light beam by a vapour-containing sample with that of a vapour-free sample of carrier gas (198.1).

b) T If a gas is passed over a heated wire, heat is lost from the wire to the gas. The rate of heat loss will depend upon the flow rate, temperature and the thermal conductivity of the gas. Cooling of the wire reduces its electrical resistance. The change can then be converted into an electrical output which is dependent upon the gas concentration. This describes the katharometer which is most commonly used to measure carbon dioxide and helium (198.1).

c) T The solubility of a vapour in rubber is the mechanism of the Dräger 'Narkotest'®. Here the instrument contains silicone rubber strips under slight tension. The absorption of a vapour into the rubber changes the tension in a concentration-dependent way (198.1).

d) T If nitrogen is subjected to high voltage (2000 V) in a gas discharge tube, then light will be emitted with concentration-dependent intensity. This instrument can be used for breath-by-breath nitrogen analysis in, for example, the assessment of closing volume (198.1).

e) T Infrared absorption by carbon dioxide is the standard method of analysis (198.1).

199 The mechanism of action of local anaesthetic agents is well described in several modern texts. The section in Dundee is recommended reading (199.1).

When a local anaesthetic is applied to a nerve fibre:
a) the inside of the cell membrane is affected by un-ionized drug
b) ionized drug causes sodium channels to close
c) the resting transmembrane potential is elevated
d) the threshold potential is unaffected
e) the rate of depolarization is slowed

200 Amyloid is a homogeneous, refractile pale pink material composed of protein fibrils. Its deposition is associated with a plethora of clinical conditions.

The following may be associated with amyloidosis:
a) nephrotic syndrome
b) restrictive cardiomyopathy
c) myeloma
d) peripheral neuropathy
e) Waterhouse–Friderichsen syndrome

References

199.1 Dundee, Clarke & McCaughey   p 283–288

200.1 Souhami & Moxham   p 1092–1093
200.2 Souhami & Moxham   p 705

199 Local anaesthetic agents cause a temporary failure of propagation of nerve impulses along any affected nerve. The applied solution is highly ionized but in equilibrium with its unionized form. The unionized portion crosses the lipoprotein cell membrane by diffusion, and another equilibrium then develops between ionized and unionized drug within the cell. It is the ionized portion of the drug which closes sodium channels on the inside of the cell membrane. This has the effect of slowing the rate of depolarization and reducing the potential reached. The resting potential and the threshold potential for propagation are not altered.

    a) F See above (199.1).
    b) T See above (199.1).
    c) F See above (199.1).
    d) T See above (199.1).
    e) T See above (199.1).

200 Amyloidosis is a generic term for a group of conditions where the tissues are infiltrated by a waxy substance which stains pink with the haematoxylin and eosin stain. The infiltrate ultimately damages tissue by pressure, atrophy or hypoxia. The reactive type of amyloidosis may occur in chronic inflammatory conditions, or in association with immunoglobulin-producing tumours.

    a) T (200.1).
    b) T (200.1).
    c) T Primary amyloid usually accompanies myeloma (200.1).
    d) T (200.1).
    e) F The Waterhouse–Friderichsen syndrome is acute adrenal destruction complicating septicaemia, usually meningococcal (200.2).

201 In the manufacture of nitrous oxide:
a) nitrogen may be a contaminant
b) the ammonium nitrate process generates heat
c) the higher oxides of nitrogen may be produced if the temperature is too low
d) potassium permanganate is used in the purification process
e) the optimum temperature for the ammonium nitrate process is 350°C

202 One of the more commonly featured statistical tests in scientific papers is the chi-squared test. It is not universally applicable and has limitations. Know them.

The chi-squared test:
a) can only be applied to a 'two-by-two' table
b) Yates' correction should be applied to small samples
c) is appropriate for continuous data
d) always shows one degree of freedom
e) may be used when the data are proportions

References

201.1 Anaesthesia Review 7   p 93–95

202.1 Swinscow   p 41–52

201 A knowledge of the processes used in the manufacture of medical gases gives an indication of the deleterious effects of contaminants. The most common process for the manufacture of nitrous oxide involves heating ammonium nitrate to the temperature at which it breaks down into nitrous oxide and water. The other oxides of nitrogen, plus nitrogen itself, may be produced as well, especially if the temperature is not properly controlled.

a) **T** Other compounds produced by the ammonium nitrate process include nitrogen, nitric acid, nitric oxide and nitrogen dioxide. The nitrogen is difficult to remove and may remain at a concentration of 0.5% (201.1).

b) **T** This process is exothermic, it produces heat. That is why the temperature in the retort is so difficult to control (201.1).

c) **F** The higher oxides tend to be produced in greater quantities if the temperature is too high (201.1).

d) **T** Potassium permanganate is used to remove nitric oxide (201.1).

e) **F** 250°C (201.1).

202 The chi-squared tests are a means of comparing the distribution of discrete variables in one sample with the distribution of discrete variables in another sample. The tests must be done on actual numbers, not percentages, proportions, means or other derived statistics.

a) **F** These tests can be done on larger tables (202.1).

b) **T** There is a school of thought which suggests that Yates' correction should be used for all 'two by two' chi-squared tests (202.1).

c) **F** See above (202.1).

d) **F** The number of degrees of freedom is determined by the minimum number of figures which must be supplied to enable the investigator to complete the whole table. There is one degree of freedom in a 'two-by-two' table, but correspondingly more in larger tables (202.1).

e) **F** See above (202.1).

203 Intestinal obstruction in infants may be associated with:
a) pyelonophritis
b) meconium ileus
c) meningitis
d) Down's syndrome
e) cystic fibrosis

204 This question assumes that all other factors are constant, such as arterial pressure and arterial partial pressure of carbon dioxide.

Cerebral blood flow may increase during anaesthesia with:
a) an infusion of a barbiturate
b) nitrous oxide
c) midazolam
d) an infusion of propofol
e) an infusion of etomidate

References

203.1 Black   p 365–370

204.1 Michenfelder   p 41
204.2 Goodman & Gilman   p 307–308
204.3 Focus on Infusion   p 162–164
204.4 Dundee, Clarke & McCaughey   p 157–165

203a) T Any cause of septicaemia in a child may also cause paralytic ileus (203.1).
  b) T Meconium ileus is one of the causes of mechanical intestinal obstruction in the neonate. There is an association with cystic fibrosis (see below) (203.1).
  c) T (203.1).
  d) T In Down's syndrome there is a high incidence of other malformations, including duodenal atresia (203.1).
  e) T An association exists between cystic fibrosis and meconium ileus (203.1). See above.

204 A complex relationship exists between the cerebral blood flow (CBF) and the cerebral metabolic rate for oxygen ($CMRO_2$). In general, anaesthesia reduces $CMRO_2$ even if there is an increase in CBF. The precise effect is agent specific but, in general, the vapours increase CBF while the intravenous agents reduce it. Candidates are recommended to read the references before attempting to answer this question. All of these agents reduce $CMRO_2$.
  a) F (204.1).
  b) T (204.1).
  c) F (204.1).
  d) F (204.2, 204.3, 204.4).
  e) F (204.1, 204.4).

205 Pharmacokinetics is the study, in mathematical terms, of the absorption, distribution and elimination of drugs from the body. These processes can be mathematically represented by a number of theoretical compartments which are interlinked in a precise way.

When a bolus intravenous injection is made:
a) after distribution, the plasma concentration will be the dose given divided by the plasma volume
b) the volume of distribution is the plasma volume
c) elimination by zero order kinetics is the most common method of excretion
d) the time constant is the time it takes for the plasma concentration to fall to half of its original level
e) the fall in plasma concentration follows an exponential curve

206 The pituitary gland has been described as the conductor of the endocrine orchestra in that, by negative feedback and the secretion of trophic hormones, it controls most functions of the endocrine system. Most of the features of global pituitary failure are those of failure of the target organs.

A patient with pituitary failure may have:
a) hyperpigmentation
b) fasting hypoglycaemia
c) reduced aldosterone secretion
d) infertility
e) loss of axillary hair

References

205.1 Dundee, Clarke & McCaughey   p 27–33

206.1 Zilva & Pannall   p 114–117

205a) F After distribution, the plasma concentration will be the dose given divided by the volume of distribution (205.1).

b) F The volume of distribution (V_d) is a theoretical volume which relates the dose given and the measured plasma concentration. V_d may be greater or less than the plasma volume depending upon whether there is active extraction from the plasma, or a high-affinity store. In the latter case, V_d may be greater than the whole body volume (205.1).

c) F Elimination by zero order kinetics presents a straight line fall in plasma concentration with time. This implies a rate limiting step of some sort, usually an enzyme process. The more common method of elimination, first order kinetics, produces an exponential fall in concentration with time, and elimination is concentration dependent (205.1).

d) F This describes half-life. The time constant is the time to reach zero concentration if the initial rate of fall of concentration were maintained from the starting level down to zero. For any uni-exponential decay, the half-life is equal to 0.698 time constants. In one time constant, the concentration will fall to 36.8% of the initial value (205.1).

e) F Drugs following first order kinetics will have a single exponential decay. Drugs with zero order kinetics (see **c**) will follow a straight line decay, whereas drugs with second or higher orders may follow multi-exponential decay curves (205.1).

206a) F The hyperpigmentation which occurs in Addison's disease (primary adrenal failure) results from high levels of adrenocorticotrophic hormone (ACTH). ACTH is not raised in pituitary failure (206.1).

b) T Because of cortisol and/or growth hormone deficiency, patients are sensitive to insulin and so may show fasting hypoglycaemia (206.1).

c) F Aldosterone is not under pituitary control (206.1).

d) T Infertility is one of the signs of gonadotrophin deficiency (206.1).

e) T Loss of secondary sexual characteristics, including loss of adult hair patterns, is a feature of gonadotrophin deficiency (206.1).

207 On a modern anaesthetic machine:
a) the audible oxygen failure warning device will be sounded by nitrous oxide
b) there will be a total gas shut-off device
c) when there is an oxygen pressure failure, the breathing system should open to atmosphere
d) there will be a pressure relief valve set at 3 bar
e) there should be a visual warning of oxygen failure

208 The respiratory quotient (RQ) is the ratio of carbon dioxide output to oxygen absorption. For carbohydrate this is 1.0, because for each molecule of oxygen used in carbohydrate metabolism, one molecule of carbon dioxide is formed. For fat and protein metabolism the RQ is lower, because a large proportion of the oxygen consumed is used to combine with the excess hydrogen ions formed.

The respiratory quotient (RQ):
a) will be low immediately after a meal
b) may be assessed accurately by measuring the respiratory exchange ratio
c) is 0.8 for protein
d) may be low in diabetes mellitus
e) will rise eight to ten hours after a meal

References	
207.1 Synopsis	p 150
208.1 Guyton	p 778–779

207a) F The oxygen failure warning device should be sounded by residual oxygen pressure in a reservoir (207.1).

b) T When oxygen pressure fails, all other gases should be cut off so that a hypoxic mixture cannot be given. This should not be confused with a fail-safe device, which it is not (207.1).

c) T There is an air entrainment valve on many machines. This may or may not be useful because, in the event of gas failure, a minute volume divider ventilator will not entrain air, and a patient breathing spontaneously may only entrain enough air into the breathing system to rebreathe to and from the reservoir bag (207.1).

d) F The usual setting for this valve is 30 kPa (0.3 bar). The valve is to protect the machine from the consequences of obstructed outlet, not to protect the patient, which falls to other devices (207.1).

e) T (207.1).

208 The maximum RQ in health is 1.0.

a) F The RQ after a meal approaches unity because most of the food consumed is carbohydrate (208.1).

b) T The respiratory exchange ratio is the output of carbon dioxide by the lungs divided by the uptake of oxygen in the same time. Over a short period, an hour or so, this will exactly equal the RQ (208.1).

c) T (208.1).

d) T In diabetes, lack of insulin prevents carbohydrate utilization and so fat and protein are used instead, lowering the RQ (208.1).

e) F About 8 to 10 hours after a meal, most of the carbohydrate stores have been used up and so the RQ falls as fat becomes the predominant substrate (208.1).

209 The plasma expanders in everyday use vary in their nature and content. Any widely used agent must be known in detail. Read the bottle labels which list the electrolytic composition.

Polygeline:
a) is a urea-linked gelatin solution
b) is presented as a 5% solution
c) has an average molecular weight of 50 000 daltons
d) contains no potassium
e) contains 5 mmol/l of calcium

210 Fat embolism is an under-diagnosed condition which may prove fatal.

Fat embolism may be associated with:
a) a long bone fracture 5–7 days previously
b) petechial haemorrhages over the upper torso
c) hypoxaemia
d) thrombocytopenia
e) dyspnoea, tachycardia and confusion

References

209.1 Data Sheet Compendium   p 570–571

210.1 Stoelting   p 192–193

209a) T Polygeline is met as Haemaccel ® — a modified and degraded gelatin with urea linkages (209.1)
   b) F It is a 3.5% solution not 5% (209.1).
   c) F The average molecular weight is 35 000 daltons (209.1).
   d) F Potassium is present at a concentration of 5.1 mmol/l (209.1).
   e) F Calcium is present at a concentration of 6.25 mmol/l (209.1).

210 Fat embolism is a common complication of bony trauma. It usually presents 12–72 hours after a long bone fracture or multiple injuries. Long bones are not __always__ involved. The presentation is of sudden onset of dyspnoea, tachycardia and confusion, with cyanosis. There may be a petechial rash over the upper body. Fat droplets may be seen in the urine and the retinal vessels, and there may be infiltrates on chest X-ray. There is a suggestion that the fat, or a breakdown product of fat, may cause a toxic capillary leakage in the pulmonary and cerebral circulations (210.1).
   a) F See above (210.1).
   b) T See above (210.1).
   c) T Hypoxaemia is not the only possible cause of the mental confusion (210.1).
   d) T Thrombocytopenia may be mild or severe (210.1).
   e) T See above (210.1).

211 Drugs from a wide range of differing groups may affect the tone of skeletal muscle. This may be an unwanted or a desired effect of a drug.

Skeletal muscle relaxation is seen with:
a) dantrolene
b) nifedipine
c) baclofen
d) enflurane
e) diltiazem

212 The Bernouilli effect is seen when a high pressure jet of gas is passed across the open end of a small tube, the other end of which is in fluid. The fall in pressure at the open end (Venturi effect) causes fluid to rise up the tube to be nebulized at the open end. There is often an anvil for the stream of droplets to impact upon, breaking them up further.

An unheated Bernouilli effect nebulizer:
a) is not affected by back pressure
b) needs a separate high pressure gas supply
c) tends to warm the carrier gas
d) is more efficient than an ultrasonic nebulizer
e) produces droplets in a narrow range of sizes

References

211.1	Dundee, Clarke & McCaughey	p 568
211.2	Dundee, Clarke & McCaughey	p 414–415
211.3	Goodman & Gilman	p 774–780
211.4	Goodman & Gilman	p 479–480
211.5	Dundee, Clarke & McCaughey	p 108
212.1	Parbrook	p 154–156

211 Muscle contraction is the end result of a long sequence of events from the brain to the actin–myosin bundle which may be interrupted at a number of sites.

a) **T** Dantrolene dissociates excitation-contraction coupling in the muscle cell by preventing the release of calcium ions from the sarooplasmic reticulum. This produces intracellular muscle relaxation (211.1, 211.2).

b) **F** (211.3).

c) **T** Baclofen is a derivative of the neurotransmitter gamma aminobutyric acid. As such, baclofen inhibits mono- and polysynaptic transmission in the spinal cord, reducing the frequency and intensity of muscle spasms after cord transection (211.4).

d) **T** Enflurane, in common with the other ether anaesthetic agents, has a direct muscle relaxant effect (211.5).

e) **F** (211.3).

212a) F Backpressure in a Bernouilli nebulizer causes a change in the difference between the carrier gas pressure and the driving gas pressure. This alters the entrainment ratio (212.1).

b) **T** See above (212.1).

c) **F** In the unheated version there is a cooling effect because some of the water vaporizes, requiring latent heat of vaporization. Heating increases the efficiency of the device (212.1).

d) **F** The ultrasonic nebulizer is more efficient than the heated Bernouilli nebulizer (212.1).

e) **F** The anvil of a Bernouilli nebulizer produces droplets of a wide range of sizes from 20 microns to 1 micron in diameter (212.1).

213 The following physical properties may be used in the measurement of pressure:
a) change of electrical resistance in a wire
b) variable inductance
c) focusing of light
d) change in flow through a narrow tube
e) Torricellian vacuum

214 Horner's syndrome comprises miosis, ptosis, enopthalmos and loss of sweating on the affected side.

A unilateral Horner's syndrome may occur:
a) as a complication of central venous catheterization
b) as a complication of subclavian perivascular local anaesthesia of the brachial plexus
c) in the treatment of quinine poisoning
d) during routine lumbar epidural anaesthesia
e) in association with vertebral artery occlusion

References

213.1   Sykes, Vickers & Hull   p 153–162
213.2   Sykes, Vickers & Hull   p 201–203

214.1   Davidson   p 866
214.2   Shoemaker   p 136–140
214.3   Nimmo & Smith   p 1077–1078
214.4   Souhami & Moxham   p 59
214.5   Morgan   p 83
214.6   Souhami & Moxham   p 896–897

213a) T The electrical resistance of a wire alters with change in tension. If the wire is bonded to a transducer diaphragm then the change in resistance can be used to measure the displacement and therefore the pressure applied to the diaphragm (213.1).

b) T If a metallic rod attached to a diaphragm is passed through a magnetic field, then the change in inductance can be used as a measure of the displacement of the diaphragm and hence the pressure (213.1).

c) T A light beam focussed upon a silvered diaphragm will change its focus with alteration of the shape of the diaphragm in response to applied pressure (213.1).

d) F The flow of a fluid through a narrow tube causes flow-dependent differences in pressure between the two ends of the tube. This, the Venturi effect, is the operating principle of the pneumotachograph. The change in pressure is used to measure the flow, not the other way round (213.2).

e) T The Torricellian vacuum is the vacuum above a mercury column in a tube sealed at the top with the open end in a pool of mercury. This is the working principle of the mercury barometer (213.1).

214 Horner's syndrome is the result of interruption of the sympathetic pathways to the head. This pathway starts in the lower brain stem, passes through the cervical cord, out to the white rami communicantes of C8 and T1 and into the lower cervical and upper thoracic sympathetic ganglia (214.1).

a) T The list of complications of central venous catheterization is endless. The stellate ganglion may be damaged by the needle used to insert the catheter, or by a haematoma which forms later or after arterial damage (214.2).

b) T Horner's syndrome is a regular feature of this technique with up to 70% incidence. Remember that 'subclavian' relates to the position of the plexus not to the approach used (214.3).

c) T Quinine poisoning causes retinal artery spasm to the extent of blindness. This has been treated by stellate ganglion block, repeated (possibly bilaterally) which causes a Horner's syndrome. Treating both sides at the same time puts the phrenic nerves and vertebral arteries at risk (214.4).

d) T Horner's syndrome may occur in relation to normal epidural anaesthesia and seems to bear no relation to the height of the block (214.5).

e) T Occlusion of the vertebral artery or the posterior inferior cerebellar artery causes infarction of the lateral medulla. The tracts involved include the sympathetics, resulting in a Horner's syndrome. There are many other signs in this condition, but all come under the heading of Wallenberg syndrome (214.6).

215 High frequency jet ventilation (HFJV):
a) cannot be used in patients with broncho-pleural fistula
b) improves carbon dioxide output in patients with adult respiratory distress syndrome (ARDS)
c) increases mean intrathoracic pressure when compared to intermittent positive pressure ventilation (IPPV)
d) works at frequencies up to 100 breaths per minute (bpm)
e) can be used with unsedated patients

216 The effects of stress, burns, injury and surgery are much the same in terms of nutrition. Protein and fat are broken down more than in the non-injured. There is a general sympathetic overactivity, including the adrenal cortex, and secretion of hormones associated with catabolism is increased.

In the metabolic response to injury there may be:
a) hypoglycaemia
b) reduced nitrogen excretion
c) resistance to the effects of insulin
d) increased secretion of glucagon
e) increased secretion of catecholamines

References	
215.1 Shoemaker	p 641–645
216.1 Shoemaker	p 1085–1093

215a) F Broncho-pleural fistula, or bronchial air leaks from any cause, are positive indications for HFJV as gas exchange can be maintained with less air leakage because of the lower intrabronchial pressures compared to IPPV (215.1).
   b) T (215.1).
   c) F Mean intrathoracic pressure is lower in HFJV than IPPV, which is one of its stated advantages (215.1).
   d) F HFJV is applied at frequencies of 60–600 bpm (215.1).
   e) T The ease of use on unsedated patients is one of the major advantages when it comes to weaning from ventilation (215.1).

216a) F Hyperglycaemia occurs due to insulin resistance (216.1).
   b) F Nitrogen excretion is increased (216.1).
   c) T see **a** (216.1).
   d) T Glucagon secretion is increased (216.1).
   e) T Catecholamine output is increased (216.1).

217 Drowning and near drowning show a variety of clinical features. The variation in physiological effects depends upon the exact circumstances of the incident.

In near drowning:
a) there may be pulmonary oedema
b) there need not be inhalation of fluid
c) there is usually hyperkalaemia
d) there may be hypovolaemia
e) cerebral hypoxia may be delayed in warm water drowning

218 When a patient presenting for emergency surgery is known to be a carrier of human immunodeficiency virus (HIV), the following precautions should be taken against cross-infection:
a) gloves need only be worn when the anaesthetist does not have intact skin
b) used needles should be carefully handed to a nurse for disposal
c) used needles should be placed in a thick cardboard disposal bin for incineration
d) eye protection is only necessary if there is a risk of substantial spillage of blood
e) tubes and equipment from the breathing system must be destroyed after use

---

References

217.1 Shoemaker   p 64–67

218.1 Nimmo & Smith   p 975–980

217 In drowning and near drowning there are differences between warm and cold water, salt and fresh water, aspiration and non-aspiration, activity or otherwise. In general, cold water drowning causes breath holding and hypothermia. This may prolong the period of survivability. Large quantities of inhaled water will alter blood volume and electrolytes, depending upon whether the water was salt or fresh.

    a) T Pulmonary oedema may be caused by the fluid shifts of water inhalation or by neurogenic mechanisms following cerebral hypoxia (217.1).

    b) T Immersion of the face in cold water causes breath holding or laryngeal spasm; thus, the victim may be hypoxic but have dry lungs (217.1).

    c) F Hypokalaemia is more usual (217.1).

    d) T The fluid shifts may result in a low blood volume, while fluid in the lungs results in oedema (217.1).

    e) F In warm water drowning, the metabolic demand for oxygen continues at a relatively normal level and hypoxia develops quickly. In cold water drowning, the body temperature falls rapidly and so does the oxygen requirement, delaying the onset of hypoxic tissue damage (217.1).

218 Health care workers are at risk from the diseases of their patients. Fortunately, across the world there are very few health professionals known to have become HIV positive in the line of duty. There are many more who have become hepatitis B positive. Precautions should be strict but, having said that, the known case is probably not the one that spreads the infection so it would be reasonable for anaesthetists to assume that all patients are potential sources.

    a) I Gloves should be worn when there is a risk of contact with <u>any</u> body fluid when the anaesthetist has scratches or other open wounds on their hands (218.1).

    b) F The number of people at risk should be minimized. Used needles should be disposed of <u>by the user</u> (218.1).

    c) F Cardboard is not substantial enough to withstand needle penetration. The bin should be metal or thick plastic (218.1).

    d) T Reference 281.1 suggests that eye protection is only necessary if significant blood spillage is anticipated. There are other fluids which contain virus and, in the authors' opinion, it would be reasonable to take precautions in anticipation of other fluids being spilled. HIV is not known to be transmitted in aerosol form (218.1).

    e) F Disposable equipment should be disposed of safely. Other equipment should be either autoclaved or cold sterilized, for example three hours in fresh glutaraldehyde (218.1).

219 Although clinically based questions such as this are often met in the examination, they are notoriously difficult to answer unequivocally

Twelve hours after a transurethral prostatectomy, a 65-year-old man becomes confused and has tachypnoea:
a) hypotension would be compatible with a diagnosis of TUR syndrome
b) a tachycardia would be compatible with a diagnosis of bacteraemic shock
c) a low central venous pressure would be compatible with a diagnosis of TUR syndrome
d) the rapid respiration suggests bacteraemia rather than TUR syndrome
e) the presence of hyponatraemia would not support the diagnosis of TUR syndrome

220 **Complications of haemorrhagic shock include:**
a) pituitary failure
b) pancreatitis
c) acute hepatic failure
d) acute tubular necrosis
e) colitis

References

219.1	Synopsis	p 482–483
219.2	Whitfield & Hendry	p 518–525
220.1	Souhami & Moxham	p 677
220.2	Surg Clin N Amer (1989) 69:3	p 467–480
220.3	Johnson & Imrie	p 311–312
220.4	Jamieson & Kay	p 483–484
220.5	Sherlock	p 116–117
220.6	Shoemaker	p 711–721
220.7	OTM	p 12.158–159

219 The facts presented in the stem of this question are unhelpful in making a diagnosis. Confusion and hyperventilation are features of both TUR syndrome and bacteraemic shock, and both of these conditions are possible after TURP. The further information in the completions is more specific.

a) F Patients with TUR syndrome tend to be hypertensive, not hypotensive (219.1).

b) T Tachycardia supports bacteraemic shock as a diagnosis. TUR syndrome tends to cause bradycardia (219.1, 219.2).

c) F TUR syndrome is caused by excessive absorption of hypotonic fluid with a low sodium concentration. There is almost inevitably a high CVP. On the other hand, patients with bacteraemic shock tend to have a low or normal CVP (219.1, 219.2).

d) F Hyperventilation does not differentiate between these two possibilities (219.1, 219.2).

e) F The presence of significant hyponatraemia would confirm the diagnosis of TUR syndrome rather than refute it (219.1, 219.2).

220 a) T This is Sheehan's syndrome of pituitary necrosis following obstetric haemorrhage (220.1).

b) F But note that reference (220.2) suggests that pancreatitis may occur after the cold, low flow perfusion of cardiopulmonary bypass. Hypovolaemia is not mentioned in the aetiology of pancreatitis in reference (220.3).

c) T As the blood pressure falls in shock, so do hepatic blood flow and oxygen consumption. After a prolonged period, acute hepatic failure may ensue (220.4, 220.5).

d) T One of the better known complications of haemorrhage. Oliguria is the presenting sign and although initially this is prerenal and reversible, it becomes irreversible unless adequate treatment is instituted (220.6).

e) T Ischaemic colitis, a necrosis of the intestinal mucosa, occasionally presents after severe shock. There is usually a history of occlusive vascular disease (220.7).

221 Concerning medical gas cylinders in the UK:
   a) an oxygen cylinder will have a grey body with black and white shoulders
   b) an air cylinder will have a black body with white shoulders
   c) a carbon dioxide cylinder will have a grey body with grey shoulders
   d) a brown body with brown and white shoulders will indicate a cylinder for an oxygen/helium mixture
   e) a blue body with blue shoulders indicates a nitrous oxide cylinder

222 When conducting a pre-use check of an anaesthetic machine:
   a) when the nitrous oxide supply is disconnected there should be a reduction in the flow of oxygen
   b) there should be no flow of nitrous oxide when the oxygen supply is disconnected
   c) the standard check gives no indication as to which gas flows through which flowmeter
   d) the pressure relief valve should operate only if the common gas outlet is completely occluded
   e) the gas hose probes should not fit into an outlet for another gas

References

221.1 Dunnill & Colvin   p 8–9

222.1 Synopsis   p 147

221 Cylinder colours should be known and recognized. Any non-standard mixtures will be clearly labelled by writing on the cylinder body. See Table 4.

   a) F Grey body with black and white shoulder designates air (221.1).
   b) F Black body with white shoulder designates oxygen (221.1).
   c) T (221.1).
   d) F For an oxygen/helium mixture, the body colour should be black, though the shoulder colour is correct (221.1).
   e) T (221.1).

Table 4 Cylinder colours

Contents	Body colour	Shoulder colour
Oxygen	Black	White
Air	Grey	Black/white
Nitrous oxide	Blue	Blue
Nitrous oxide/oxygen mixture	Blue	Blue/white
Carbon dioxide	Grey	Grey
Carbon dioxide/oxygen mixture	Black	Grey/white
Helium	Brown	Brown
Helium/oxygen mixture	Black	Brown/white

222a) F A reduction in the flow of oxygen when the nitrous oxide is turned off suggests that there is nitrous oxide leakage into the oxygen pipework (222.1).
   b) T Modern machines should have a total gas shut-off device so that no other gases can flow when the oxygen has failed (222.1).
   c) T The only true way to establish which gas flows through which flowmeter is by the use of a gas analyser (222.1).
   d) T Only with complete occlusion should the pressure within the pipework reach the limits necessary to blow off the relief valve (222.1).
   e) T The probes and the internal sizes of the collars should be gas specific (222.1).

223 Retinoblastoma is a rare malignant tumour of the retina (1 in 20 000 live births) which presents in childhood.

Retinoblastoma:
a) exists in both hereditary and non-hereditary forms
b) is associated with osteosarcoma
c) lymphatic spread is common
d) is resistant to radiotherapy
e) lung metastases are common

224 Sodium nitroprusside:
a) causes smooth muscle relaxation mediated by alpha adrenergic neurones
b) depresses myocardial contractility
c) causes rebound hypertension when administration of the drug is stopped
d) causes methaemoglobinaemia
e) reduces platelet aggregation

References

223.1 Pediatric Opthalmology   p 348–364

224.1 Dundee, Clarke & McCaughey   p 386–390

223 There seems to be a dichotomy in the formation of retinoblastoma. The presence of a single genetic mutation is essential but only causes a predisposition to the tumour. A second mutation is necessary for tumour growth. This second mutation may be in the germinal cell, in which case both retinae of the affected child may have tumour, or the second mutation may be in the retinal cell itself in which case only one retina will be affected (223.1).

a) **T** The genetics explained above indicates that when the mutation is in the germinal cell there will be inheritance, and where it is in the retinal cells there will not (223.1).

b) **T** The hereditary form is associated with other, extra-orbital malignant tumours, including osteosarcoma (223.1).

c) **F** Lymphatic spread only occurs if extra-orbital tissues are invaded (223.1).

d) **F** Fortunately for the affected children, this tumour is very radiosensitive (223.1).

e) **F** Lung metastases are very rare. Metastasis to other sites – bone, marrow, liver – is more common (223.1).

224 Sodium nitroprusside is a direct acting smooth muscle relaxant which is metabolized to cyanide and thiocyanate by enzymes present in liver and kidney. The toxic effects are upon the cytochrome system. The recommended dose is up to 10 μg/kg per min by intravenous infusion.

a) **F** The drug acts directly, not via a nerve pathway (224.1).

b) **F** Cardiac function is maintained or increased unless the preload is significantly reduced by excessive dosage (224.1).

c) **T** Rebound hypertension can be a problem, especially after neurosurgery (224.1).

d) **T** Nitroprusside is broken down to nitrite and cyanide. The nitrite combines with haemoglobin to produce methaemoglobin and then, after cyanide release, cyanmethaemoglobin (224.1).

e) **T** At doses greater than 3 μg/kg per min there is an inhibition of platelet aggregation and an increase in the bleeding time (224.1).

225 Dental anaesthesia has been carried out in dental surgeries for years but there have been reported deaths. Dentists and dental anaesthetists are now subject to constraints, following the publication of the Poswillo report.

The Expert Working Party on General Anaesthesia, Sedation and Resuscitation in Dentistry recommends that:
a) sedation be used in preference to general anaesthesia whenever possible
b) for sedation by inhalation the minimum concentration of oxygen be fixed at 50%
c) any technique of sedation should have a margin of safety wide enough to render unintentional loss of consciousness unlikely
d) flumazenil should be used routinely for termination of benzodiazepine sedation
e) an electrocardiogram, pulse oximeter and non-invasive blood pressure device are recommended whenever general anaesthesia is used

226 Since the explosive anaesthetic agents fell into disuse, the antistatic precautions in operating theatres have become less rigid. They are, however, still important in the construction and use of the theatre suite.

With regard to antistatic precautions in operating theatres:
a) an electrically conductive floor is necessary
b) the electrical resistance of rubber wheels should be as low as possible
c) cotton clothing should have conductive strips
d) footwear with a leather sole is acceptable
e) the zone of risk is 25 cm from the patient breathing system

References

225.1 Poswillo Report

226.1 Synopsis   p 97–98

225 The Expert Working Party which produced this report took into consideration all aspects of dental anaesthetic practice. In outline, the Working Party is suggesting that all dental sedation and anaesthesia should be carried out by properly trained anaesthetists in properly equipped premises with appropriately trained ancillary staff and to the highest standards of hospital practice.

a) T Sedation is recommended over general anaesthesia (225.1).
b) F The minimum recommended oxygen concentration is 30% (225.1).
c) T This is a counsel of perfection (225.1).
d) F Flumazenil should be available but only used in an emergency (225.1).
e) F The report states 'essential' (225.1).

226 Antistatic precautions may seem to be obsolete, but they are still required in the construction of theatres.

a) T The floor should conduct electricity but with a moderate resistance so that static and conventional electricity do not have an alternative path to earth (226.1).
b) F The resistance of rubber wheels should be between 50 kilohms and 10 megohms/cm^2 so as to provide a route to earth of medium resistance (226.1).
c) F Cotton clothing is the ideal because it is not subject to static discharges. There is no requirement for conduction (226.1).
d) T (226.1).
e) T Diethyl ether and cyclopropane are little used now and so this is largely irrelevant (226.1).

227 Dental anaesthesia is renowned for the frequency with which arrhythmias are encountered. Many research hours have been put into the consideration of how they may be prevented or reduced.

The incidence of cardiac arrhythmias during general anaesthesia for dental extraction may be reduced by:
a) infiltration with local anaesthetic
b) beta blockade
c) using enflurane rather than halothane
d) administration of atropine
e) intravenous rather than inhalational induction

228 The hydroxyethyl starches are recent additions to the list of available plasma expanders. Refer to question 132.

Solutions of hydroxyethyl starch:
a) are presented in saline solution
b) decrease the erythrocyte sedimentation rate
c) will expand the plasma volume, pentastarch more than the same volume of hetastarch
d) are predominantly eliminated by hepatic metabolism
e) have a pH in the physiological range

References

227.1 Churchill-Davidson   p 1131–1132

228.1 Data Sheet Compendium   p 427
228.2 Data Sheet Compendium   p 435

227 Most of the abnormal rhythms are ventricular or nodal, but seem to be benign in that they have little or no effect on perfusion or cardiac output and return to sinus rhythm at the end of the procedure. It has been suggested that these disturbances may be the cause of the occasional death.

a) T Local anaesthesia reduces but does not abolish the problem (227.1).

b) T Beta blockade may be effective but is impractical, especially in children, and may cause other problems instead, bradycardia for example (227.1).

c) T Halothane gives a 25% incidence of arrhythmia, enflurane less so. Unfortunately, enflurane is not at all easy to use in the dental chair (227.1).

d) F Atropine doubles the incidence of halothane induced arrhythmia (227.1).

e) T (227.1).

228a) T Sodium concentration is 154 mmol/l for both solutions (228.1, 228.2).

b) F ESR is increased, not decreased. This can be employed usefully in the centrifugal collection of granulocytes (228.1).

c) T Pentastarch expands circulating volume by 1.5 times the expansion of hetastarch (228.2).

d) F Most excretion of the hydroxyethyl starches is renal (228.1, 228.2).

e) F The pH of Hespan® (hetastarch) is 5.5 approximately, while that of Pentaspan® (pentastarch) is 5.0 approximately (228.1, 228.2).

229 Candidates should have some knowledge of methods of sterilization and disinfection of equipment, especially of which methods are suitable for which materials.

When equipment is sterilized or disinfected:
a) soaking in chlorhexidine and alcohol for 30 minutes will kill all vegetative bacteria and all spores
b) repeated ethylene oxide exposure will damage polyvinyl chloride (PVC) equipment
c) soaking in 2.5% glutaraldehyde for 30 minutes will kill all vegetative bacteria and some spores
d) repeated gamma irradiation of PVC causes no damage to it
e) an autoclave routine of 3 minutes at 134°C and 221 kPa (32 lb/in^2) will be adequate for most equipment

230 The differentiation between upper and lower motor neurone lesions merely requires the application of basic physiology.

In the presence of an upper motor neurone lesion:
a) muscle bulk will be reduced
b) muscle tone will be reduced
c) plantar responses will be flexor
d) reflexes will be increased
e) coordination may not be impaired

References

229.1 Churchill-Davidson   p 1188–1191

230.1 Souhami & Moxham   p 873

229 Disinfection is the removal of vegetative organisms while spores may survive. Sterilization is the removal of all organisms and spores.
 a) F Soaking in a mixture of chlorhexidine and alcohol kills bacteria but not spores (229.1).
 b) F Ethylene oxide appears not to damage PVC on repeated sterilization. This method is used widely for initial sterilization of disposable equipment, because heat damages PVC. Ethylene oxide is not used much for repeat sterilization because the process involves prolonged leaching and bacteriological testing, all of which extends the turn-round time (229.1).
 c) T Glutaraldehyde (Cidex)® will not kill all spores (229.1).
 d) F Repeated gamma irradiation makes PVC both discoloured and brittle. This method is not in regular use for repeat sterilization (229.1).
 e) T This is the standard regimen for rubber anaesthetic equipment (229.1).

230 Examination of the nervous system provides basic clinical information. In general, an upper motor lesion will cause increased tone, increased reflexes, extensor plantars and a spastic gait with normal muscle bulk. Power is usually reduced, and sometimes coordination is impaired. A lower motor neurone lesion will cause fasciculation with reduced tone, power and reflexes, impaired coordination and reduced muscle bulk (230.1).
 a) F See above (230.1).
 b) F See above (230.1).
 c) F See above (230.1).
 d) T See above (230.1).
 e) T See above (230.1).

231 Polycythaemia is characterized by an increase in the number of circulating red cells. It follows that the haematocrit will be raised.

Polycythaemia rubra vera may be associated with:
a) thrombocytopenia
b) increased tissue oxygen delivery
c) gout
d) splenomegaly
e) leukocytosis

232 Despite its long history, the pathophysiology of Guillain-Barré syndrome (GBS) is still not fully understood.

The Guillain-Barré syndrome (acute inflammatory polyneuropathy) may be associated with:
a) autonomic involvement
b) 10–200 cells per mm^3 of cerebrospinal fluid
c) bilateral facial weakness
d) a good response to steroid treatment
e) complete recovery in more than 95% of patients

References

231.1 Souhami & Moxham   p 1074–1076

232.1 Souhami & Moxham   p 941
232.2 Davidson   p 986–987

231 Polycythaemia rubra vera (PRV) is a malignant myeloproliferative disorder, a result of an increased sensitivity to erythropoietin. Increased <u>production</u> of erythropoietin produces <u>secondary</u> polycythaemia not PRV. Despite its name, PRV is not confined to the red cell.

a) F Thrombocytosis is the rule; indeed, it is one of the diagnostic criteria (231.1).

b) F While the red cell mass and the haemoglobin concentration may increase, the blood viscosity also increases in line with these, reducing blood flow to tissues and thus oxygen delivery (231.1).

c) T Gout occurs because of the increased erythropoietic activity (231.1).

d) T 75% of patients with PRV are said to have splenomegaly (231.1).

e) T Leukocytosis is also one of the diagnostic criteria, showing PRV to be a condition of the multipotential haemopoietic stem cell rather than the red cell line itself (231.1).

232 The Guillain-Barré syndrome is one of those conditions which, though said to be rare, turn up with regularity in intensive care units. Commonly, a patient with GBS is presented with a view to respiratory support because of deteriorating pulmonary function. The diagnosis is not always made in advance of admission.

a) T Although the condition is usually motor and sensory, autonomic involvement is common enough to be a problem (232.1).

b) F The cellularity of the CSF in GBS is usually normal. Cellularity of this level (10–200/mm^3) would indicate that an acute infective process was involved, poliomyelitis for example (232.1).

c) T Bilateral facial weakness is a common sign of GBS (232.1, 232.2).

d) F The response to steroids is very poor (232.1, 232.2).

e) F 80% of patients make a complete recovery, 10% have residual weakness which may be significant, and 10% die (232.2).

233 The proportion of the population over 70 years of age is increasing rapidly, along with the number of surgical procedures carried out on them.

When comparing men over 70 years of age with their younger counterparts:
a) plasma cholinesterase concentrations are lower in the elderly
b) there is increased lung compliance in the elderly
c) thiopentone has an increased volume of distribution in the elderly
d) there is increased chest wall compliance in the elderly
e) there is reduced ability to retain sodium in the elderly

234 A steady-state blood concentration of a drug:
a) will be achieved in two elimination half-lives if a single speed infusion is used
b) will be achieved most rapidly by using a bolus dose, an infusion which reduces exponentially, and a maintenance infusion at the same time
c) could be achieved in a one-compartment model by a bolus equal to the steady state concentration times the volume of distribution, followed by a single speed maintenance infusion
d) can be maintained by an infusion at the steady state concentration times the drug clearance
e) will follow an exponential decay when administration is stopped if first order kinetics apply

References

233.1 Miller   p 1969–1979

234.1 Dundee, Clarke & McCaughey   p 32–33
234.1 Calvey & Williams   p 42–47

233a) T The stem specifies that <u>men</u> are under consideration. Plasma cholinesterase concentrations are lower in geriatric men than in geriatric women or in the young of either sex, though why this should be so is unclear (233.1).

  b) T Lung compliance is increased because of the loss of elastin and elastic recoil. Chest wall compliance and total compliance are not under consideration in this completion (233.1).

  c) F Thiopentone has a decreased volume of distribution in the elderly, resulting in higher plasma concentrations and greater effect for the same dose (233.1).

  d) F Chest wall compliance is decreased in the elderly. This, combined with the increase in lung compliance (see **b**) means that total compliance changes very little. (233.1).

  e) T Reduced ability to retain sodium is part of the change in renal structure and function with age. There is also a reduced response to antidiuretic hormone (233.1).

234 The pharmacokinetics of infusions are not easily understood. Interpatient variability is wide.

  a) F A constant infusion will achieve steady state concentrations in between four and five elimination half-lives, not two, and the concentration will follow a rising exponential curve (234.1, 234.2).

  b) T This method will give a steep rise from zero concentration to the steady state with no overshoot. Pumps which produce this profile are available but of limited use because of the complicated mathematics necessary to produce the desired plasma concentration (234.1, 234.2).

  c) T While this may be true, the desired steady state concentration and the volume of distribution of likely drugs are not usually tip-of-the-tongue knowledge for most of us (234.1, 234.2).

  d) T (234.1, 234.2).

  e) T As with bolus doses, the plasma concentration will fall exponentially if first order kinetics apply. This does not imply that biological effect will decay similarly (234.1, 234.2).

235 Factors affecting the activity of plasma cholinesterase have obvious practical significance, especially with regard to the use of suxamethonium.

The usual form of plasma (pseudo) cholinesterase is inhibited by:
a) pancuronium
b) cinchocaine
c) prednisolone
d) amethocaine
e) 0.05 mmol/l sodium fluoride

236 The chemoreceptor trigger zone (CTZ) is responsible for the mediation of the sensation of nausea. Many antiemetic agents affect this area.

The chemoreceptor trigger zone is affected by:
a) chlorpromazine
b) haloperidol
c) apomorphine
d) tetrahydrocannabinol
e) domperidone

References

235.1 Bowman   p 228–230

236.1 Dundee, Clarke & McCaughey   p 239–254
236.2 Goodman & Gilman   p 924–926

235 Plasma cholinesterase has no known natural function, and absence or limited activity seems not to be detrimental to health. In the anaesthetic situation, this enzyme is important in the breakdown of the ester local anaesthetics and some other unrelated drugs, including suxamethonium. The activity of the enzyme may be altered by the presence of yet more drugs or by medical conditions such as hepatic or renal disease.

a) T Apparently so (235.1).

b) T Cinchocaine is also known as dibucaine and is used in the assessment of cholinesterase activity in the laboratory. Cinchocaine at a concentration of 0.01 mmol/l will inhibit the usual form of enzyme by more than 70% of its activity (235.1).

c) F Prednisolone reduces hepatic production of the enzyme, not its activity (235.1).

d) T Amethocaine is an ester local anaesthetic which inhibits the enzyme. It is also a substrate for pseudocholinesterase (235.1).

e) T Part of the laboratory test for cholinesterase activity. Sodium fluoride at this concentration inhibits the normal enzyme by about 64% of its activity. The other variants of the enzyme are inhibited to different degrees by this concentration of fluoride (235.1).

236a) T The phenothiazines mostly have H_1 antihistamine effects, and are effective as antiemetics at the CTZ. The associated sedation may limit their usefulness in the treatment of motion sickness (236.1).

b) T (236.1).

c) T Apomorphine is an agonist at the CTZ, and has been used both for induced vomiting and for experimental testing of antiemetics (236.2).

d) T Tetrahydrocannabinol, an extract from cannabis, is an extremely potent antiemetic, effective even against cancer chemotherapy agents (236.2).

e) T (236.1).

237 There has been a great deal of interest in prognosis/severity scoring. There is still no good indicator of survival potential with universal application.

In the APACHE II disease severity classification system:
a) total scores below 20 indicate poor outcome
b) previously documented disease is not considered
c) a score is taken directly from the Glasgow Coma Scale
d) scores for pre-existing disease differ between emergency and elective admissions
e) age carries no additional score if the patient is otherwise healthy

238 The described functions of opioid receptors change frequently, as does their classification, making the framing of meaningful questions very difficult. There may be subpopulations of each receptor with different affinities for agonists and antagonists.

At the mu opioid receptor:
a) cholecystokinin may be an agonist
b) hallucinations are an agonist response
c) miosis is an agonist response
d) dependence is not an agonist response
e) dynorphin is a potent agonist

References

237.1 Shoemaker   p 1452–1453

238.1 Dundee, Clarke & McCaughey   p 203–206

237 The APACHE (Acute Physiology and Chronic Health Evaluation) scoring system gives a more scientific indication of prognosis in acutely ill patients than clinical impression alone. There are always problems with rigid scoring systems and this is no exception. Points are added for deviation from the normal range in 11 physiological or biochemical areas — arterial pH, serum sodium, creatinine, Pa_{O_2} or A-a oxygen difference and so on — and also for the Glasgow coma scale (15 points minus actual coma scale). To this is added a score for age (up to 45 years = 0, 45–54 years = 2, 55–64 years = 3, 65–74 years = 5, over 75 years – 6 pts) and further points are added for documented pre-existing severe disease such as portal hypertension, cirrhosis, COPD, renal and cardiovascular disease in the New York Heart Association class IV group. More points are added for emergency admissions in each of the chronic disease groups than for elective admission. A score of 25 points suggests a 50% in-hospital mortality, rising to 90% at more than 40 points.

a) F See above (237.1).
b) F See above (237.1).
c) T See above (237.1).
d) T See above (237.1).
e) F See above (237.1).

238a) F Cholecystokinin seems to be an antagonist at the mu receptor, possibly involved in the termination of agonist effect (238.1).
b) F Hallucination is an agonist response, but at the sigma receptor not the mu receptor (238.1).
c) T Miosis is an agonist effect at mu and kappa receptors but not at sigma (238.1).
d) F Dependence is an agonist effect (238.1).
e) F Dynorphin is a potent agonist but at the kappa receptor sites, not mu (238.1).

239 Polyuria is an increase in the <u>volume</u> of urine produced, not an increase in the frequency of voiding.

Polyuria may be associated with:
a) chronic renal failure
b) obstructive uropathy
c) hypokalaemia
d) propranolol
e) lithium therapy

240 The bleeding time is a scientific measure of both platelet and capillary integrity and function. It takes practice, however, to get reproducible results.

The bleeding time is not usually prolonged with:
a) thiazide diuretics
b) von Willebrand's disease
c) a platelet count greater than 100 000 mm^3
d) chronic renal failure
e) acute alcohol intoxication

References

239.1	Davidson	p 553
239.2	Souhami & Moxham	p 799–816
239.3	Goodman & Gilman	p 420–421
239.4	Goodman & Gilman	p 231
240.1	OTM	p 19.220–231
240.2	Davidson	p 750–751

239a) T Chronic renal failure is not a single disease and oliguria is not a universal feature. There are forms of renal failure where the kidney fails to concentrate or otherwise modify the glomerular filtrate. A high osmotic load from urea may cause polyuria (239.1, 239.2).

  b) T Obstructive uropathy causes a secondary renal medullary dysfunction so that water and sodium are not reabsorbed and polyuria results (239.1, 239.2, 239.3).

  c) T Acquired nephrogenic diabetes insipidus results in failure of sodium reabsorption, which causes potassium depletion due to the secondary diuresis (239.1, 239.2).

  d) F Propranolol reduces renal blood flow and glomerular filtration rate because of a fall in cardiac output (239.1, 239.4).

  e) T Lithium is handled by the kidney in a similar way to sodium. The extra solute load on the kidney may cause polyuria (239.1, 239.3).

240 Read the question. 'NOT usually prolonged with'.
  Because of the wording of the stem this question becomes difficult. If the wording were 'may be associated with ' it would be straightforward.

  a) F The thiazides depress thrombopoiesis by interfering with megakaryocyte maturation (240.1).

  b) F Von Willebrand's disease is both a capillary fragility problem and a failure of platelet aggregation. The platelets themselves are not defective but there is an absence of a plasma factor responsible for inter-platelet bridging (the von Willebrand factor) (240.1).

  o) T An increase in bleeding time with normally functioning platelets tends to occur with platelet counts below 100 000/mm^3, although some references suggest 30 000/mm^3 as the lower limit for normal function (240.1, 240.2).

  d) F In chronic renal failure, the bleeding time is prolonged because of the production of abnormal platelet forms (240.1).

  e) F In both acute and chronic alcohol intoxication (even with normal liver function) there is a platelet-related increase in bleeding time. The production of platelets is supressed and the pre-existing platelets are prevented from aggregation (240.1).

241 The outputs of transducer measuring systems, especially when used for invasive measurement of vascular pressure, are subject to influences other than that of the patient's blood pressure. Calibration and frequency response are of paramount importance.

In a measuring system consisting of a transducer and fluid filled catheter:
a) the resonant frequency will be highest with a stiff transducer and a narrow-bore catheter
b) the best frequency response is produced when there is critical damping
c) critical damping is the situation when there is no overshoot after a step change in applied pressure
d) inadequate damping will produce a waveform with high-frequency distortion of the signal
e) alterations in damping will alter the measured mean of a waveform

242 The term 'Mendelson's syndrome' is better avoided because of ambiguity regarding its meaning. To some it is aspiration per se, to others it is the resulting picture, major lung dysfunction.

Pulmonary aspiration of gastric contents in late pregnancy may be associated with:
a) bronchospasm
b) a low alveolar-arterial gradient for oxygen
c) hypovolaemia
d) metabolic acidosis
e) necrosis of alveolar type I cells

References

241.1 Sykes, Vickers & Hull   p 166–173

242.1 Morgan   p 214

241a) F The highest resonant frequency occurs with a stiff transducer and a wide-bore catheter because the resonant frequency is highest when the velocity of fluid movement is least, i.e. in a wide-bore catheter (241.1).

b) F Critical damping (see also **c**) is the amount of damping needed to just prevent overshoot after a step change in applied pressure. For the best frequency response in a system, this is too much. Optimum damping (64% of critical) yields the best frequency response (241.1).

c) T See **b** (241.1).

d) T Inadequate damping allows the system to oscillate at high frequency, causing distortion in the waveform (241.1).

e) F Alterations in damping will change the frequency response and the measured amplitude of the waveform, but the mean of the variable measured will not change (241.1).

242 Mendelson's syndrome was originally described in 1946 as a nonlethal complication of mask and ether anaesthesia in pregnancy. Since then it has become a less common but more lethal problem. There have been suggestions that there is a critical pH of stomach contents above which there will not be a problem, and critical volumes of gastric juice. The particulate antacids served to confuse the issue for some years, but practice has now changed in favour of H_2 receptor antagonists and non-particulate antacids.

a) T Bronchospasm is one of the more common features of the syndrome (242.1).

b) F The alveolar–arterial oxygen difference is large, not small (242.1).

c) T (242.1).

d) T Although respiratory acidosis might be expected, metabolic acidosis is often encountered (242.1).

e) T The alveoli fill with a protein-rich haemorrhagic fluid, the alveolar type I cells undergo necrosis, and the small pulmonary arterioles thrombose (242.1).

243 Glaucoma frequently requires surgical intervention. A knowledge of the aetiology may prove useful.

Glaucoma may be:
a) congenital
b) secondary to the superior vena caval syndrome
c) open angle
d) a complication of neurofibromatosis
e) traumatic

244 The wording of the stem describes the anterior approach to blockade of the sciatic nerve.

Local anaesthesia of the sciatic nerve at the level of the lesser trochanter of the femur will cause:
a) anaesthesia over the medial aspect of the knee joint
b) weakness of the quadriceps muscle
c) foot drop
d) weakness of the hamstring muscles
e) anaesthesia over the popliteal fossa

References		
243.1 Duane & Jaeger, vol 3: Ch 42	p 6	
244.1 Gray	p 1140–1149	
244.2 Wildsmith	p 158–163	

243 Glaucoma is persistently raised intraocular pressure. The consequences of untreated glaucoma are optic cupping and, eventually, blindness from optic disc compression. The causes, though many, all cause either increased production or limited drainage of aqueous humour, whether by anatomical or physiological means. The medical treatment of glaucoma may be of interest to anaesthetists. All of these completions are true.

a) **T** (243.1).

b) **T** There is high venous pressure which prevents drainage of aqueous humour (243.1).

c) **T** Primary open angle glaucoma is the most common form in adults (243.1).

d) **T** (243.1).

e) **T** Trauma may cause either inflammatory reactions in the anterior chamber or bleeding with subsequent organization of the clot (243.1).

244a) F This area is supplied (variably) by the cutaneous branch of the obturator nerve, the medial cutaneous nerve of the thigh or the saphenous nerve. None of these are branches of the sciatic (244.1, 244.2).

b) **F** The quadriceps are supplied by the femoral nerve, not the sciatic (244.1, 244.2).

c) **T** The common peroneal is a branch of the sciatic, arising above or in the popliteal fossa. It supplies the peroneal muscles which elevate the foot (244.1, 244.2).

d) **T** The hamstrings (biceps, semitendinosus and semimembranosus) are supplied by branches of the sciatic nerve below the point in question (244.1).

e) **T** The skin over the popliteal fossa is supplied by the posterior cutaneous nerve of the thigh. While this nerve is not strictly a branch of the sciatic, it runs with the sciatic in the buttock and upper thigh and so is usually blocked at the same time (244.1, 244.2).

245 The Wheatstone bridge is one of the most basic electrical measurement systems. Read about it before attempting this question

The Wheatstone bridge circuit:
a) can be used to measure changes in resistance
b) is insensitive to small changes in resistance
c) cannot be used for capacitative elements
d) gives a non-linear output
e) depends upon the ratio of the two resistances in one limb of the circuit compared to the ratio of the two resistances in the other limb

246 Ohm's law:
a) can only be applied to direct current circuits
b) can be used to derive the power of a circuit
c) suggests that resistances in parallel are additive
d) suggests that the current in a circuit is proportional to the ratio of resistance to potential difference
e) suggests that the potential differences across each of two resistors in a circuit will be in the same proportion as their resistances

References	
245.1 Sykes, Vickers & Hull	p 42
246.1 Sykes, Vickers & Hull	p 31–32

245 The Wheatstone bridge depends on simple proportions. If there are two resistances in each of the two limbs of a circuit, R1 and R2 in one limb and R3 and R4 in the other with the output ends of R2 and R4 connected together, and a current measuring device, M, connected between the halfway points of each limb, then there will be no current through M if the ratio R1:R2 is the same as R3:R4. If there is a small change in one of the resistances there will be a large but non-linear change in the current flow through M. This device can be used to measure an unknown resistance if the other three are known, or if one is unknown and another variable but known. This principle can also be applied to capacitance and reactance (245.1).
  a) **T** (245.1).
  b) **F** (245.1).
  c) **F** (245.1).
  d) **T** (245.1).
  e) **T** (245.1).

246 Ohm's law will be familiar from schooldays. It is:

$$E = IR$$

where E is the potential difference, I the current flowing and R the resistance. Also written as I=E/R. When resistances are in series then they are additive; when they are in parallel then the combined resistance Rt may be assessed by 1/Rt = 1/R1 + 1/R2 where R1 and R2 are two resistances in parallel.
  a) **F** Alternating current circuits can be assessed just as well (246.1).
  b) **T** The power in Watts (joule-seconds) is given by W = I E , (power = current times potential difference). If two of the current, resistance or potential difference are known, then the other element and the power follow by simple calculation (246.1).
  c) **F** see above (246.1).
  d) **F** The stem indicates that I=R/E when in fact I=E/R (246.1).
  e) **T** The current in a circuit must be the same at all points. As I = E/R then E1/R1 must be the same as E2/R2, though this completion is a longwinded way of saying it (246.1).

247 Enzyme induction follows prolonged administration of a variety of substances, and can be a problem if the handling of drugs is affected by the induced enzymes. The enzymes concerned are those in the microsomal oxidative and reductive pathways.

Hepatic enzyme induction is seen with:
a) propranolol
b) cimetidine
c) phenytoin
d) diazepam
e) halothane

248 The clearance of a drug:
a) has the units 'mass per unit time'
b) is the volume of plasma completely emptied of drug in unit time
c) relates only to metabolism by one organ
d) is not directly related to the plasma concentration of the drug
e) is not the same as the extraction ratio

References

247.1	Calvey & Williams	p 24–25
247.2	Dundee, Clarke & McCaughey	p 403–408
247.3	Goodman & Gilman	p 239
247.4	Goodman & Gilman	p 353–354
248.1	Calvey & Williams	p 39–42
248.2	Dundee, Clarke & McCaughey	p 31–32

247a) F Propranolol is not known to be an enzyme-inducing drug. The availability of propranolol may be reduced because its metabolism is increased when other drugs have caused enzyme induction (247.2, 247.3).
 b) F Cimetidine inhibits microsomal liver enzymes (247.1).
 c) T Phenytoin is one of the best known enzyme inducers (247.1).
 d) F Diazepam and the other benzodiazepines do not cause liver enzyme induction (247.4).
 e) T Halothane, enflurane and methoxyflurane are known to induce liver enzymes, mostly after long exposure (247.1).

248 Clearance is a useful pharmacological concept. It is defined as the volume of plasma completely cleared of drug in unit time and can be applied to individual organs or to the body as a whole. The units are volume cleared per unit time, and thus it is independent of plasma concentration. The classical method, using urine, is to collect urine over a period and divide the total amount of drug eliminated in that time by the area under the plasma concentration–time curve for the same period (248.1, 248.2).
 a) F The units are volume per unit time, not mass per unit time (248.1).
 b) T See above (248.1, 248.2).
 c) F See above. This can be used for the whole body or for several organs summatively (248.1, 248.2).
 d) T Because the clearance is volume cleared per unit time, the plasma concentration itself is not used. The area under the plasma concentration–time curve may, however, be used (248.1, 248.2).
 e) T The extraction ratio is the proportion of drug which is removed in one passage through the relevant organ. It is not the clearance (248.2).

249 Helium is an inert gas with applications in anaesthetic practice.

Helium:
a) has a low density compared to air
b) has a high viscosity compared to air
c) will improve gas flow if flow is laminar
d) makes turbulent flow less likely
· e) has a low thermal conductivity

250 Consider carefully the qualifying word 'commonly' in the stem.

Haemoptysis is commonly associated with:
a) Wegener's granulomatosis
b) mitral stenosis
c) bronchiectasis
d) systemic lupus erythematosus
e) pulmonary metastases

References		
249.1	Nunn	p 47–51
249.2	Nunn	p 328
250.1	Souhami & Moxham	p 512
250.2	Souhami & Moxham	p 458

249a) T (249.1).
  b) F The viscosity of helium is similar to air (249.1).
  c) F The resistance to flow during laminar flow is dependent more on the viscosity than the density (249.1).
  d) T The change from laminar to turbulent flow depends upon the ratio of density to viscosity. Helium, being less dense, reduces the resistance during turbulent flow but also makes turbulent flow less likely (249.1).
  e) F Helium has a high thermal conductivity, which makes hypothermia more likely when it is used for diving (249.2).

250a) T Wegener's granulomatosis is a vasculitis mainly of the upper respiratory tract and kidney (250.1).
  b) T (250.2).
  c) T (250.2).
  d) T The features of systemic lupus erythematosus include pulmonary vasculitis which leads to haemoptysis (250.2).
  e) F Haemoptysis is unusual with pulmonary metastases but common with primary lung cancers and pulmonary tuberculosis (250.2).

251 Prolonged action of non-depolarizing muscle relaxants may be encountered in the viva section of the examination under the guise of 'failure to reverse'.

Prolonged action of non-depolarizing neuromuscular blocking agents may be associated with:
a) hypocalcaemia
b) respiratory acidosis
c) metabolic alkalosis
d) frusemide
e) hypomagnesaemia

252 Calf muscle pain on exercise may be caused by:
a) McArdle's disease
b) spinal stenosis
c) isolated stenosis in the profunda femoris artery
d) phosphofructokinase deficiency
e) syringomyelia

References

251.1	Dundee, Clarke & McCaughey	p 275–277
251.2	Dundee, Clarke & McCaughey	p 301
251.3	Miller	p 418–426
252.1	Davidson	p 831
252.2	Souhami & Moxham	p 930–934
252.3	Gray	p 783–784

251a) T Acetyl choline release in response to depolarization can be inhibited either by a reduction in the extracellular concentration of calcium or by an increase in the extracellular concentration of magnesium. The reduction in acetyl choline release will reduce competition for receptor sites and prolong the action of the muscle relaxant (251.1).

b) T This effect is probably related to the acidosis caused but is not consistent between relaxants (see **c**)(251.2).

c) T Metabolic alkalosis also prolongs neuromuscular blockade so, in view of **b**, this cannot be entirely related to pH but must be related to the effect of acid-base changes on other electrolytes (251.3).

d) T Even a single dose of frusemide seems to have a presynaptic inhibitory effect on acetylcholine release, intensifying and prolonging neuromuscular blockade (251.3).

e) F Hypermagnesaemia prolongs and intensifies neuromuscular blockade. Hypomagnesaemia is not known to do so (251.3).

252a) T McArdle's disease is a muscle glycogen storage disease with deficiency of the myophosphorylase enzyme. The result is pain on exercise and increased glycogen deposition. Eventually there is muscle wasting (252.1).

b) T Spinal canal stenosis presents with ischaemic nerve entrapment signs on exercise, including pain, numbness and paraesthesia in the legs (252.2).

c) F The profunda femoris supplies the muscle of the thigh. The completion states 'isolated', so candidates cannot invoke vascular disease of the main femoral artery to make this completion true (252.3).

d) T Phosphofructokinase deficiency presents in a similar way to McArdle's disease (252.1).

e) F Syringomyelia has a variable presentation, in common with all the demyelinating diseases. The main features are a dissociated loss of pain and temperature sensation, usually proximally first but eventually leading to a spastic paraplegia. Pain sensation is lost (252.2).

253 Epilepsy comprises a group of conditions in which there are recurring episodes of altered cerebral function associated with paroxysmal excessive discharge of cerebral neurones.

The following drugs may be used in the treatment of epilepsy:
a) ethosuximide
b) primidone
c) clonazepam
d) carbamazepine
e) phenytoin

254 Clinical features of disturbance in potassium regulation are a frequent examination topic. There is a paucity of revision material. Reference 254.1 is recommended.

The following may be seen in hypokalaemia:
a) weakness
b) muscle pain
c) peaked T waves on ECG
d) cardiac arrhythmias
e) diarrhoea

References	
253.1 Davidson	p 858
254.1 Zilva & Pannall	p 62

253a) T Ethosuximide is particularly useful for the treatment of petit mal 'absence' type of seizures (253.1).
  b) T Primidone is used for the treatment of grand mal tonic-clonic seizures (253.1).
  c) T Clonazepam, a benzodiazepine drug, is indicated for the treatment of partial type seizures. Sedation is a profound side effect (253.1).
  d) T Carbamazepine is used for the treatment of both tonic-clonic and partial seizures (253.1).
  e) T Phenytoin remains the most widely prescribed of the anti-epileptic agents (253.1).

254a) T Weakness results from derangement of neuromuscular transmission and is often accompanied by painful muscle cramps, particularly in the chronic situation (254.1).
  b) T See above (254.1).
  c) F Peaked T waves are a classic feature of <u>hyper</u>kalaemia.
  d) T Cardiac arrhythmias are commonly seen in hypokalaemic states (254.1).
  e) F Diarrhoea is not a feature of hypokalaemia, though prolonged or severe diarrhoea may itself cause hypokalaemia (254.1). Be wary of confusing these two, different, situations.

255 In gout, urate crystals are deposited in various tissues — joints, tendon sheaths, kidney and urinary tract. The urate is derived from purine metabolism, originally from nucleic acids. The deposition of the poorly soluble urate may result from high production, reduced solubility or reduced excretion.

Gout may be associated with:
a) gastrointestinal haemorrhage
b) aspirin
c) hypomagnesaemia
d) glucose-6-phosphatase deficiency
e) psoriasis

256 Plasma urea concentration below the normal range may be associated with:
a) starvation
b) the polyuric phase of acute renal failure
c) pregnancy
d) chronic liver disease
e) an inborn error of metabolism

References

255.1	Davidson	p 795–798
255.2	Zilva & Pannall	p 379–387
256.1	Zilva & Pannall	p 13–18
256.2	Zilva & Pannall	p 367

255a) T In gastrointestinal bleeding from whatever cause there is a large blood 'meal' in the digestive tract. The excessive purine metabolic load as this is digested causes a rise in urate synthesis with no accompanying increase in excretion (255.1, 255.2).

b) T Aspirin causes a change in urate solubility by altering the acid–base state (255.1, 255.2).

c) F Hypomagnesaemia is associated with chondrocalcinosis (pyrophosphate arthropathy), not gout (255.1).

d) T Patients with G-6-P deficiency have both increased purine metabolism and reduced renal urate excretion because of their lactic acidosis (255.1, 255.2).

e) T Gout occurs in conditions of increased purine turnover, such as psoriasis (255.1, 255.2).

256 Urea is an hepatic product of protein and amino acid metabolism. The normal kidney has a large capacity for excretion.

a) F In starvation there is a change from predominantly carbohydrate metabolism to protein-based metabolism. Because of the increase in protein turnover in starvation, the urea concentration increases (256.1).

b) F In the oliguric phase of renal failure, urea accumulates and is excreted during the polyuric phase. The plasma concentration does not fall below normal (256.1).

c) T The plasma urea concentration falls in pregnancy because of haemodilution and an increase in glomerular filtration rate (256.1).

d) T The failing liver cannot metabolize amino acids and proteins and so the production of urea is reduced. There is also a dilutional effect (256.1).

e) T There is an inborn error of the urea cycle where ammonia cannot be converted to urea (256.1, 256.2).

257 Nalorphine proved to be useful as an agent for reversing the effects of opioids. Later derivatives of 'purer' antagonist effect included naloxone and naltrexone.

Naloxone:
a) is the n-allyl derivative of morphine
b) has a longer terminal half-life than morphine
c) has a low lipid solubility
d) does not cross the placenta to any significant degree
e) does not increase blood pressure unless an opioid has been used

258 Naltrexone:
a) is an opioid agonist
b) has a shorter half-life than naloxone
c) has a high bioavailability
d) reverses morphine analgesia
e) may be given orally

References

257.1 Dundee, Clarke & McCaughey   p 221–228
257.2 Dundee, Clarke & McCaughey   p 525
257.3 Goodman & Gilman   p 515

258.1 Goodman & Gilman   p 514–516

257a) F Naloxone is the n-allyl derivative of oxymorphone, not morphine (257.1).
  b) F Naloxone has a terminal half-life shorter than most of the opioids in current use (257.1).
  c) F High lipid solubility (257.1).
  d) F The placental transfer of naloxone is good enough for maternal administration to antagonize fetal intrauterine respiratory depression (257.2).
  e) T The outpouring of catecholamines and rise in blood pressure which follows administration of naloxone tends only to occur after prior administration of opioids, unless the dose of naloxone is in excess of 0.3 mg/kg (257.1,257.3).

258a) F Naltrexone is one of a family of opioid antagonists which were developed after the introduction of naloxone. Others in this group include naloxazone (which binds extremely tightly to receptors) and nalmefene (258.1).
  b) F Naltrexone has a much longer half-life than naloxone — around three hours (258.1).
  c) T The bioavailability of naltrexone is greater than that of naloxone. The drug is liver metabolized to 6-naltrexol (258.1).
  d) T This is true of any opioid antagonist (258.1).
  e) T Naltrexone may be given by both parenteral and oral routes (258.1). The drug was originally developed for use in opioid dependency states.

259 The myocardium may be affected in:
   a) Duchenne muscular dystrophy
   b) facio-scapulo-humeral muscular dystrophy
   c) dystrophia myotonica
   d) myotonia congenita
   e) Charcot-Marie-Tooth disease

260 Malignant hyperpyrexia (MH) is exceedingly rarely met in practice (incidence about 1 in 200 000 patients). Its frequency in examinations is greater. No apologies are made for a second question in this volume. Refer to question 26.

   Malignant hyperpyrexia may be associated with:
   a) atrophy of the quadriceps femoris muscle
   b) kyphosis
   c) osteogenesis imperfecta
   d) Duchenne muscular dystrophy
   e) dystrophia myotonica

References

259.1	Stoelting	p 622–625
259.2	Stoelting	p 323
260.1	Stoelting	p 857–861
260.2	Stoelting	p 623–625

259 Conditions which affect skeletal muscles may also affect myocardium. This is not, however, universally applicable.
   a) T (259.1).
   b) F (259.1).
   c) T (259.1).
   d) F (259.1).
   e) F Charcot-Marie-Tooth disease is a neurological condition which causes atrophy of the peroneal muscles. There is no apparent myocardial involvement (259.2).

260 Malignant hyperpyrexia is an hereditary muscle condition which has associations with other muscle conditions. The presence of one of these conditions should raise the anaesthetist's awareness that MH is a possibility.
   a) F The myopathy of MH includes <u>hyper</u>trophy of the quadriceps rather than atrophy (260.1).
   b) T Conditions which show imbalance of muscles may also have an association with MH (260.1).
   c) T Osteogenesis imperfecta is associated with MH (260.1).
   d) T Duchenne type muscular dystrophy is associated with MH (260.1, 260.2).
   e) T Dystrophia myotonica is associated with MH (260.1).

261 The most famous of the mucopolysaccharidoses is undoubtedly Hurler's syndrome, otherwise known as 'gargoylism'. The group also contains Hunter's syndrome.

Hurler's syndrome:
a) is a glycogen storage disease
b) is accompanied by skeletal dysplasia
c) mental function is normal
d) is inherited as a Mendelian dominant
e) is accompanied by corneal clouding

262 The following are found in Marfan's syndrome:
a) aortic stenosis
b) lens dislocation
c) arachnodactyly
d) recessive inheritance
e) mitral valve prolapse

References

261.1 Souhami & Moxham   p 782
261.2 Davidson   p 808–809

262.1 Davidson   p 807

261a) F Hurler's syndrome is not a glycogen storage disease, but one of the mucopolysaccharidoses. This family of genetic disorders involves the metabolism of glycosaminoglycan, resulting in multiple sites of substrate deposition accompanied by various clinical features (261.1, 261.2).
  b) T Skeletal dysplasia is a feature of both Hurler's and Hunter's syndromes (261.2).
  c) F The norm is gross mental retardation (261.1).
  d) F The inheritance of Hurler's syndrome is autosomal recessive (261.2).
  e) T Corneal clouding is a feature of the syndrome (261.1, 261.2).

262a) F It is aortic incompetence which is seen in Marfan's syndrome (262.1).
  b) T Dislocation of the lens occurs in sufferers (262.1).
  c) T Arachnodactyly and high arched palate are two cardinal clinical signs of Marfan's syndrome (262.1).
  d) F Marfan's syndrome is inherited by phenotypically heterogeneous dominant transmission (262.1).
  e) T Mitral valve prolapse is a feature of the condition (262.1).

263 Rheumatoid arthritis is the commonest form of chronic inflammatory joint disease with a prevalence among Caucasians of 1%. The disease affects many other organ systems apart from the musculoskeletal.

Features of rheumatoid lung include:
a) fibrosing alveolitis
b) pleural effusion
c) pulmonary nodules
d) Felty's syndrome
e) Caplan's syndrome

264 The most frequently encountered disease produced by a mycobacterium is tuberculosis. In general, the mycobacteria are responsible for a wide variety of clinical conditions including the major third world disease, leprosy.

Mycobacteria may cause:
a) pneumothorax
b) pleurisy
c) diabetes mellitus
d) lymphadenopathy
e) ulceration of the lower limbs

References

263.1 Davidson   p 762–771
263.2 Souhami & Moxham   p 514

264.1 Davidson   p 364–365
264.2 Souhami & Moxham   p 280

263a) T Fibrosing alveolitis is, however, one of the rarer features of rheumatoid lung (263.1).
  b) T Pleural effusions occur in 1% of sufferers of rheumatoid arthritis (263.1).
  c) T Nodularity on chest X-ray is frequently seen in rheumatoid lung. This is one of the features of Caplan's syndrome (263.2).
  d) F Felty's syndrome comprises splenomegaly, neutropenia and rheumatoid arthritis. The syndrome of rheumatoid lung is that of Caplan (263.1, 263.2).
  e) T See above. Caplan's syndrome comprises nodular change in the lung fields, positive anti-nuclear factor and rheumatoid arthritis (263.2).

264a) T It is the rupture of a primary tuberculous complex which is usually responsible for the sudden development of pneumothorax (264.1).
  b) T Pleurisy is a common association of pulmonary tuberculosis. Pleural pain may also result from pneumothorax (264.1).
  c) F None of the mycobacterial illnesses will directly cause diabetes mellitus.
  d) T Lympadenopathy is common in mycobacterioses. It is particularly marked in tuberculosis (264.1).
  e) T *Mycobacterium ulcerans* infection results in ulcers on the lower limbs (264.2).

265 Atropine:
  a) is prepared as a racemic mixture
  b) is *dl* hyoscyamine
  c) is an isomer of hyoscine
  d) has antimuscarinic activity in the *d* form
  e) depresses the reticular activating system

266 Lactic acid is harmless per se. The acidosis induced by it may cause severe metabolic problems.

  Lactic acidosis may be associated with:
  a) insulin-dependent diabetes mellitus
  b) von Gierke's disease
  c) impaired hepatic gluconeogenesis
  d) glibenclamide
  e) metformin

References

265.1	Dundee, Clarke & McCaughey	p 318–323

| 266.1 | Zilva & Pannall | p 206–208 |
| 266.2 | Dundee, Clarke & McCaughey | p 499–501 |

265a) T Atropine is *dl* hyoscyamine (see **b**), a racemic mixture of the two optical isomers (265.1).
  b) T see **a** (265.1).
  c) F Hyoscine and atropine are the scopine and tropine esters, respectively, of tropic acid. Scopine has an oxygen bridge between carbons 6 and 7 in the base whereas tropine does not. Otherwise the molecules are identical (265.1).
  d) F Only the laevorotatory (*l*) form has antimuscarinic activity (265.1).
  e) T Atropine has a number of cerebral effects. Depression of the reticular activating system is one such (265.1).

266a) T Diabetic ketoacidosis includes an element of lactic acidosis (266.1).
  b) T Patients with von Gierke's disease, glucose-6-phosphatase deficiency, tend to develop lactic acidosis (266.1).
  c) T Hepatic and renal gluconeogenesis (sourced from lactate) are aerobic processes. They cannot therefore occur anaerobically and so, in the face of poor tissue oxygenation, lactate accumulates instead of being converted to glucose (266.1).
  d) F The sulphonylureas do not cause lactic acidosis; the biguanides do (see **e**) (266.2).
  e) T Metformin and phenformin are the drugs most notorious for causing lactic acidosis (266.1).

267 From the early understanding that the receptor system of the adrenergic system could be divided into subtypes of alpha and beta, has sprung a wealth of detail concerning the actual structure and function of each receptor subtype.

With regard to the adrenoceptors:
a) beta receptors affect G inhibitory proteins
b) beta 1, 2 and 3 types exist
c) alpha receptors stimulate adenylate cyclase
d) alpha 1 and 2 types exist
e) beta receptors stimulate adenylate cyclase

268 Pieces of equipment are often presented to candidates in the viva part of the examination. For obvious reasons, the smaller and more portable items are preferred. It is thus common to receive filters for discussion. There is a lack of revision material in textbooks. Reference 268.1 will prove invaluable.

Blood filters:
a) always have a pore size of 20 μ
b) do not remove white cells
c) are always depth filters
d) are always screen filters
e) trap microaggregate debris

References	
267.1 Goodman & Gilman	p 108–112
268.1 BJ IV Therapy (1981)	p 24–38
268.2 Anaesthesia (1985) 40	p 334–347

267a) T The beta adrenergic receptors stimulate adenylate cyclase, but this effect is mediated via the G protein known as G_s (stimulatory) (267.1).
  b) T There are now known to be subtypes 1, 2 and 3 of the beta adrenoceptor. The third subtype is 10 times more sensitive to noradrenaline than to adrenaline and is thought to mediate catecholamine responses in tissues with variable adrenergic innervation, such as adipose tissue (267.1).
  c) F The alpha adrenoceptors inhibit adenyl cyclase by an effect associated with G_i (inhibitory) protein (267.1).
  d) T Alpha adrenoceptor subtypes 1 and 2 (presynaptic) coexist (267.1).
  e) T Beta adrenoceptors stimulate adenylate cyclase in the manner described above (267.1).

268a) F The recommended filter pore size is 20–40 µ. This contrasts with the standard giving set filter pore size of 170 µ (268.1, 268.2).
  b) T Under normal circumstances, the removal of white cells by blood filters is negligible (268.1). Note, however, that artificial aggregation of granulocytes induced by spinning may result in filtration removal because large clumps are formed.
  c) F Several types of blood filter are available. Generally the most commonly used types are screen filters, but depth filters also exist as do types which combine both methods together (268.1).
  d) F See above (268.1, 268.2).
  e) T One of the major purposes in the filtration of transfused blood is the removal of microaggregate debris which is composed of fibrin, degenerate platelets, red cell debris, and fragmented granulocytes (268.1).

269 Huntingdon's chorea and Friedreich's ataxia have been deliberately paired in the last two questions. Confusion between the clinical features of these two conditions is common, and to aid clarity of thought the completions for both stems are the same.

Huntingdon's chorea:
a) is recessively inherited
b) is accompanied by dementia
c) develops under 30 years of age
d) is accompanied by cardiomyopathy
e) is accompanied by diabetes

270 Friedreich's ataxia:
a) is recessively inherited
b) is accompanied by dementia
c) develops under 30 years of age
d) is accompanied by cardiomyopathy
e) is accompanied by diabetes

References

269.1 Souhami & Moxham   p 904

270.1 Souhami & Moxham   p 924

269a) F Huntingdon's chorea is a dominantly inherited condition comprising choreiform movements and progressive dementia (269.1).
  b) T The dementia is steadily progressive from the onset of the disease. Death occurs within five years (269.1).
  c) F The usual age of onset lies between 30 and 50 years of age (269.1).
  d) F Cardiomyopathy is not associated with Huntingdon's chorea, in contrast to Friedreich's ataxia (269.1).
  e) F In contrast, a small number of patients with Friedreich's ataxia develop diabetes mellitus (see below) (269.1).

270a) T Friedreich's ataxia is inherited as an autosomal recessive condition (270.1).
  b) F Although some sufferers are said to be of limited intelligence, dementia is not part of the disease (270.1).
  c) T The ataxic element of Friedreich's ataxia is usually seen in childhood and not later than 25 years of age, in contrast to Huntingdon's chorea (see above) (270.1).
  d) T Cardiomyopathy is common (60% of patients) and usually death results in the fourth decade of life or thereabouts from cardiac failure (270.1).
  e) T Some 10% or so of sufferers develop diabetes mellitus (270.1). The reason for this is not clear.

Bibliography

The bibliography provides the key to the shortened references used throughout the book. The shortened title used in the text forms the first line of each section below and this is followed by the full reference.

AITKENHEAD & SMITH
Aitkenhead A R, Smith G (eds) 1990 Textbook of Anaesthesia, 2nd edn.
Churchill Livingstone, Edinburgh

ANAESTHESIA
Morgan M (ed) Anaesthesia (The Journal of the Association of Anaesthetists of Great Britain and Ireland). Academic Press, London

ANAESTHESIA REVIEW
Kaufman L (ed) 1982 Anaesthesia review.
Churchill Livingstone, London

ANESTHESIOLOGY
Saidman L J (ed) Anesthesiology (The Journal of the American Society of Anesthesiology Inc.) J B Lippincott Company, Philadelphia

ARCHIV FÜR KLINISCHE CHIRUGERIE
Bier A 1908 Arch. Klin. Chir. 86:1007

BOWMAN
Bowman W C 1990 Pharmacology of neuromuscular function, 2nd edn.
Wright, Bristol

BJA
Smith G (ed) British Journal of Anaesthesia. Professional and Scientific Publications, London

BJ IV THERAPY
Lowe G D 1981 Filtration in intravenous therapy:
A review of the clinical and technical aspects of intravenous fluid and blood filtration, in four parts. Part IV: Blood filters. British Journal of Intravenous Therapy, Medical Tribune Group, London

BLACK
Black J A 1987 Paediatric emergencies, 2nd edn. Butterworths, London

BMJ
Smith R (ed) British Medical Journal. British Medical Association, London

BRAUNWALD
Braunwald E (ed) 1988 Heart disease: A textbook of cardiovascular medicine, 3rd edn. W B Saunders Company, Philadelphia

BNF
British National Formulary 1991 British Medical Association and The Royal Pharmaceutical Society of Great Britain, London

BULLOCK, SIBLEY & WHITAKER
Bullock N, Sibley G, Whitaker R 1988 Essential urology. Churchill Livingstone, Edinburgh

CALVEY & WILLIAMS
Calvey T N, Williams N F 1990 Principles and practice of pharmacology for anaesthetists, 2nd edn. Blackwell Scientific Publications, Oxford

CHURCHILL-DAVIDSON
Churchill-Davidson H C (ed) 1984 A practice of anaesthesia, 5th edn. Year Book Medical Publishers Inc. Chicago

DATA SHEET COMPENDIUM
ABPI Data Sheet Compendium 1991–1992 Datapharm Publications Ltd, London

DAVIDSON
Edwards C R W, Boucher I A D (eds) 1991 Davidson's principles and practice of medicine, 16th edn. Churchill Livingstone, Edinburgh

DAVENPORT
Davenport H W 1974 The ABC of acid-base chemistry, 6th edn. The University of Chicago Press, Chicago

de GRUCHY
Firkin F C, Chesterman C N, Pennington D G, Rush B M 1989 de Gruchy's clinical haematology in medical practice, 5th edn. Blackwell Scientific Publications, Oxford

DIPRIVAN®
ICI Pharmaceuticals (UK) 1988 Diprivan — a versatile intravenous anaesthetic. ICI Pharmaceuticals (UK), Macclesfield

DUANE & JAEGER
Duane T D, Jaeger E A (eds) 1987 Clinical opthalmology. Harper and Row, Philadelphia

DUNDEE, CLARKE & McCAUGHEY
Dundee J, Clarke K, McCaughey W 1991 Clinical anaesthetic pharmacology.
Churchill Livingstone, Edinburgh

DUNNILL & COLVIN
Dunnill R P H, Colvin M P 1989 Clinical and resuscitative data, 4th edn.
Blackwell Scientific Publications, Oxford

ERIKSSON
Eriksson E (ed) 1979 Illustrated handbook in local anaesthesia, 2nd edn. Lloyd
Luke, London

FOCUS ON INFUSION
Prys-Roberts C (ed) 1991 Focus on infusion − intravenous anaesthesia.
Current Medical Literature Ltd, London

GANONG
Ganong W F 1991 Review of medical physiology 15th edn. Appleton Lange,
London.

GILES
Cushieri A, Giles G R, Moossa A R 1988 Essential surgical practice, 2nd edn.
Wright, Bristol

GOODMAN & GILMAN
Goodman G A, Rall T W, Nies A S, Taylor P 1990 Goodman and Gilman's
The pharmacological basis of therapeutics, 8th edn. Pergamon Press,
Oxford

GRAY
Williams P L, Warwick R, Dyson M, Bannister L H (eds) 1989 Gray's anatomy,
37th edn. Churchill Livingstone, Edinburgh

GRAINGER & ALLISON
Grainger R G, Allison D J (eds) 1992 Diagnostic radiology 2nd edn. An
Anglo-American textbook of imaging. Churchill Livingstone, Edinburgh

GUYTON
Guyton A C 1991 Textbook of medical physiology, 8th edn. W B Saunders
Company, Philadelphia

JOHNSON & IMRIE
Johnson C D, Imrie C W 1991 Pancreatic disease: progress and prospects.
Springer-Verlag, London

JAMIESON & KAY
Ledingham I McA, MacKay C (eds) 1988 Jamieson and Kay's Textbook of
surgical physiology, 4th edn. Churchill Livingstone, Edinburgh

HARPER
Martin D W, Mayes P A, Rodwell V W, Granner D K 1990 Harper's Review of biochemistry, 20th edn. Prentice-Hall International Inc., London

INT J OBS ANES
Reynolds F, Dewan D M (eds) 1991 International Journal of Obstetric Anesthesia. Churchill Livingstone, London

JONES
Jones P F 1987 Emergency abdominal surgery, 2nd edn. Blackwell Scientific Publications, Oxford

KAPLAN
Kaplan J 1991 Thoracic anaesthesia, 2nd edn. Churchill Livingstone, London

KATZ & KADIS
Katz J, Benumof J, Kadis L B 1990 Anesthesia and uncommon diseases, 3rd edn. W B Saunders Company, Philadelphia

MACINTOSH
Lee J A, Atkinson R S, Watt M J 1985 Sir Robert Macintosh's Lumbar puncture and spinal analgesia intradural and extradural, 5th edn. Churchill Livingstone, Edinburgh

MACLEOD
Macleod J, Munro J 1986 Clinical examination, 7th edn. Churchill Livingstone, Edinburgh

MILLER
Miller R D (ed) 1990 Anaesthesia, 3rd edn. Churchill Livingstone, Edinburgh

MICHENFELDER
Michenfelder J D 1988 Anesthesia and the brain. Churchill Livingstone, New York

MORGAN
Morgan B (ed) 1987 Foundations of obstetric anaesthesia. Farrand Press, London

MOIR
Moir D D, Thorburn J 1986 Obstetric anaesthesia and analgesia, 3rd edn. Baillière Tindall, London

MUIR
Anderson J R (ed) 1985 Muir's Textbook of pathology, 12th edn. Edward Arnold, London

NIMMO & SMITH
Nimmo W S, Smith G (eds) 1990 Anaesthesia. Blackwell Scientific Publications, Oxford

NUNN
Nunn J F 1987 Applied respiratory physiology, 3rd edn. Butterworths, London

OTM
Weatherall D J, Ledingham J G G, Warrell D A 1987 Oxford textbook of medicine, 2nd edn. Oxford University Press, Oxford

PARBROOK
Parbrook G D, Davis P D, Parbrook E O 1990 Basic physics and measurement in anaesthesia. Butterworth Heinemann, Oxford

PEDIATRIC OPTHALMOLOGY
Taylor D (ed) 1990 Pediatric opthalmology. Blackwell Scientific Publications, Boston

PED CLIN N AM
Martin L J (ed) 1987 Pediatric Clinics of North America. W B Saunders Company, Philadelphia

POSWILLO REPORT
Poswillo D E (Chairman) 1990 General anaesthesia, sedation and resuscitation in dentistry. Report of an Expert Working Party. HMSO, London

PRACTICAL PAED PROBLEMS
Hutchisson J H, Cockburn F 1986 Practical paediatric problems, 6th edn. Lloyd Luke, London

PRESCRIBER'S JOURNAL
Shenton D (ed) Prescriber's Journal. HMSO, London

RANG & DALE
Rang H P, Dale M M 1991 Pharmacology, 2nd edn. Churchill Livingstone, Edinburgh

RECENT ADVANCES
Atkinson R S, Adams A P (eds) Recent advances in anaesthesia and analgesia. Churchill Livingstone, Edinburgh

RECOMMENDATIONS FOR STANDARDS OF MONITORING
Adams A P (Chairman) 1988 Recommendations for standards of monitoring during anaesthesia and recovery. The Association of Anaesthetists of Great Britain and Ireland, London

REPORT ON CONFIDENTIAL ENQUIRIES INTO MATERNAL DEATHS
Department of Health 1991 Report on confidential enquiries into maternal deaths in the United Kingdom 1985–1987. HMSO, London

ROWLANDS
Rowlands D J 1982 Understanding the electrocardiogram. Sections 1, 2 & 3. Imperial Chemical Industries, Macclesfield

SCURR, FELDMAN & SONI
Scurr C, Feldman S, Soni N (eds) 1990 Scientific foundations of anaesthesia, the basis of intensive care. Heinemann Medical Books, London

SHERLOCK
Sherlock S 1989 Diseases of the liver and biliary system, 8th edn. Blackwell Scientific Publications, Oxford

SHOEMAKER
Shoemaker W C, Ayres S, Grenvik A, Holbrook P R, Leigh Thompson W 1989 Textbook of critical care. W B Saunders, Philadelphia

SOAP
Survey of anaesthetic practice 1988 Association of Anaesthetists of Great Britain and Ireland, London

STOELTING
Stoelting R K, Dierdorf S F, McCammon R L 1988 Anesthesia and co-existing disease, 2nd edn. Churchill Livingstone, New York

SYNOPSIS,
Atkinson R S, Rushman G B, Alfred Lee J 1987 A synopsis of anaesthesia, 10th edn. Wright, Bristol

SOUHAMI & MOXHAM
Souhami R L, Moxham J 1990 Textbook of medicine. Churchill Livingstone, London

SWINSCOW
Swinscow T D V 1982 Statistics at square one, 7th edn. British Medical Association, London

SYKES
Sykes W S 1960 Essays on the first hundred years of anaesthesia. Churchill Livingstone, London

SYKES, VICKERS & HULL
Sykes M K, Vickers M D, Hull C J 1991 Principles of measurement and monitoring in anaesthesia and intensive care, 3rd edn. Blackwell Scientific Publications, Oxford

SURG CLIN N AM
Reber H A (ed) 1989 Surgical Clinics of North America: The pancreas 69:3. W B Saunders Company, Philadelphia

TINKER & ZAPOL
Tinker J, Zapol W M (eds) 1992 Care of the critically ill patient, 2nd edn. Springer Verlag, London

TRANSFUSION
UK Department of Health 1989 Handbook of transfusion medicine. HMSO, London

TRENDS
Delarue N, Eschapasse H 1985 Trends in general thoracic surgery, vol 1. W B Saunders Company, Philadelphia

VICKERS, MORGAN & SPENCER
Vickers M D, Morgan M, Spencer P S J 1991 Drugs in anaesthetic practice, 7th edn. Butterworth Heinemann, Oxford

WALL & MELZACK
Wall P D, Melzack R (eds) 1989 Textbook of pain, 2nd edn. Churchill Livingstone, Edinburgh

WARD
Davey A J, Moyle J T B, Ward C S 1992 Ward's Anaesthetic equipment, 3rd edn. W B Saunders Company, London

WEST
West J B 1990 Respiratory physiology – the essentials, 4th edn. Williams and Wilkins, Baltimore

WHITBY, SMITH & BECKETT
Whitby L G, Smith A F, Beckett G J 1988 Lecture notes on clinical chemistry, 4th edn. Blackwell Scientific Publications, Oxford

WHITFIELD & HENDRY
Whitfield H N, Hendry W F (eds) 1985 Textbook of genitourinary surgery. Churchill Livingstone, Edinburgh

WILDSMITH
Wildsmith J A, Armitage E N 1987 Principles and practice of regional anaesthesia. Churchill Livingstone, Edinburgh

ZILVA & PANNALL
Zilva J F, Pannall P R, Mayne P D 1988 Clinical chemistry in diagnosis and treatment, 5th edn. Edward Arnold, London

Index